THE HAPPY VULVA

HOW TO ♡ YOUR DOWN-UNDER

DR FRANCES DARCY-TEHAN

First published by Ultimate World Publishing 2021
Copyright © 2021 Frances D'Arcy-Tehan

ISBN

Paperback: 978-1-922714-41-1
Ebook: 978-1-922714-42-8

Cover design: Ultimate World Publishing
Layout and typesetting: Ultimate World Publishing
Editor: Isabelle Russell
Book cover and illustrations: Cooper Jones – koops.jones@gmail.com

Ultimate World Publishing
Diamond Creek,
Victoria Australia 3089
www.writeabook.com.au

ULTIMATE WORLD
PUBLISHING

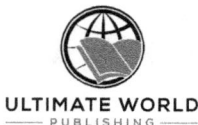

TESTIMONIALS

The Happy Vulva is an approachable and educational book about female genitalia and an indispensable resource for any woman anxious about her vulva and vagina and considering female genital cosmetic surgery. It offers helpful guidelines not just for intimacy, but for body loving.

Lindy McDougall, Macquarie University, author of *The Perfect Vagina: Cosmetic Surgery in the Twenty-First Century*

The Happy Vulva is funny, gentle and extremely informative. An exposé of industries profiteering off women's violated body image. A must-read for all women who want a healthy relationship with their down-under.

Jane Whitmore, counselling psychologist

It is very reassuring to know that there are health professionals like Dr Fran who are monitoring and caring about the sexual health and wellbeing of women.

Charmaine Morse, counselling psychologist

An informative, empathic and humorous perspective on an area of women's health and body image that remains largely underexplored. A must-read for all women.

Dr Jo Phillips, clinical psychologist

Acknowledgement Of Country

I acknowledge the Traditional Owners of the land, the Wadawurrung people of the Kulin Nation where I work and live. I pay my respects to their Elders, past, present and emerging. I celebrate the stories, culture and traditions of Aboriginal and Torres Strait Islander Elders of all communities who also work and live on this land.

DEDICATION

I dedicate this book to four mighty warrior women:

Isabella, Julia, Lucia and Teresa.

Every niece should have a crazy aunt who writes about vulvas.

THE HAPPY VULVA

How to Love Your Down-Under

This book is for all women who own a *vulva*.

The Happy Vulva will explore ways you can become your own *Vulva Image Warrior* by:

- Increasing your confidence through health literacy by expanding your *V-Knowledge* about vulval anatomy and sexual functioning.

- Empowering you to have conversations with others with your newfound *V-Knowledge*.

- Improving your sexual self-esteem and confidence about your body both in and out of the bedroom.

The Happy Vulva

How to Love Your Down-Under

Improving women's sexuality by increasing awareness of normal and natural genital diversity.

Introduction 1

V-SECTION ONE
Your Amazing Vulva

V-SECTION THREE
The Ugly Truth About Female Genital Cosmetic Surgery

V-SECTION FOUR
Vulva Victory

INTRODUCTION

As a psychologist, I was very curious as to why women who had perfectly normal genitalia would choose to undergo alteration of their genital appearance through cosmetic surgery. Women would tell me in my consultation room that they were distracted by worries about the appearance of their vulva while making out with their partner or during sexual activity. Some women were so worried about their vulval appearance or about their sexual performance that they would dread their partner making sexual overtures. For other women, they would avoid sex altogether because they thought something was wrong with them – that their vulva looked ugly. The worries or distractions about their genitalia would interfere with their ability to remain erotically focused during sexual activity. Whilst others were so worried about their genital image, they would experience sexual pain or discomfort during sexual activity. Yet, other women had difficulty having sexual penetration of the vagina because of the stress of having sexual intercourse.

As a social scientist, I wanted to understand why young girls and women were becoming anxious about the appearance of their genitals. More directly, I wanted to understand why some would desire and actually undergo unnecessary and potentially risky cosmetic surgery on their normal and healthy genitalia. I soon discovered that this area of women's sexual health and wellbeing had been severely neglected. Through my research and years of clinical practice, I have helped women learn how to improve their sexual self-esteem and experience more comfort during sexual activity.

This book draws upon my extensive clinical experience and aims to help women become more informed and confident in understanding their *down-under*. Equipped with this understanding it is hoped that women will be more confident about their body and genitals both in and out of the bedroom.

V-SECTION ONE

Your Amazing Vulva

They are like snowflakes... every one is unique and beautiful.
– Betty Dodson

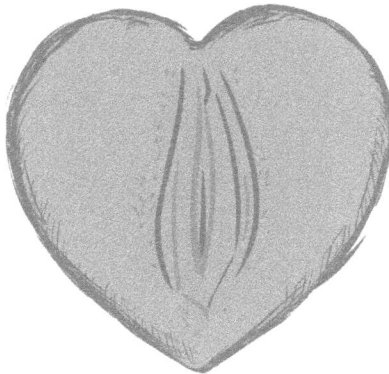

WHY SHOULD I CARE ABOUT UNDERSTANDING MY GENITALS?

Understanding your amazing vulva will increase your sexual health literacy. You will get to understand how elaborate your vulva is as you get to know its many components. Learning more about this incredible sex organ will help you to be happier and more positive about your genital appearance. This newfound confidence will also in turn, improve your sexual self-confidence both in and out of the bedroom. Pinpointing the name and location of your different *bits* will help you to clearly explain to your doctor any concerns you may have.

Understanding your genital anatomy will help you to better understand your body. Most sex tips we get are about how to seduce, please and satisfy men and we receive very little valid information in the media about women's sexual pleasure. To be a good lover is to first know and understand your own body. You may not have received the information in *The Happy Vulva* from your peers, your mother or your lover.

Learning about your genital anatomy will help you to reach your full sexual potential.

To achieve genital image positivity, it is important to understand what each part of the vulva does. By exploring your genital anatomy and describing the fascinating role they play in female sexual functioning, you will feel more empowered about your sexual self. In this chapter, I will be concentrating on the different vulval components that can be altered through cosmetic surgery. The *hymen/vaginal corona, G-spot* and *vagina* are not visible but are mentioned here as they are also subject to alteration through cosmetic surgery.

The word vagina has been commonly used to describe the vulva – it is not incorrect to call your vulva your *vagina*. It has been called many other names such as *pussy, fanny* and *vajayjay.* The term vagina has been used synonymously with vulva for a long time. However, for purposes of clarity when reading *The Happy Vulva,* I will be calling the vulva the *vulva* and the vagina the *vagina.* Using their correct anatomical names will bring us to a better understanding of our bodies and our sexual selves. *The Happy Vulva* concentrates on the wonders of your amazing vulva.

VULVA-SELFIE TOUR – A VULVA EXPEDITION

FROM YOUR MOUNTAIN TO YOUR VALLEYS (AND EVERYTHING IN BETWEEN)

Our genitals go everywhere with us, yet we know barely anything about them. At each stop of the *Vulva-Selfie Tour*, you will visit those parts of your genitals that are closest to your clothes. We are going to have a conversation about your genitals at each location. You will soon discover the many wondrous things about your vulva. You will also appreciate the special talents your vulvar parts possess and the important role they play in forming female sexuality.

Your vulva consists of all the external organs you can see outside your body and includes: the *mons pubis, labia majora, labia minora, clitoris, urethral opening, vaginal opening, vulva vestibule* and *perineum*. On this tour you will also be exploring the wonders of *pubic hair*. The *anus* will be there too as this is also a feature of your down-under landscape.

On this *Vulva-Selfie Tour* you will also journey to the vagina and paying particular attention to the *vaginal corona*, formerly known as the *hymen* and the *mystical* G-spot. They are coming along on this anatomical adventure as they are also parts of the female genitalia that can be altered through female genital cosmetic surgery.

It is important to examine yourself in order to know your true self. Doing a *Vulva-Selfie Tour* is a fantastic physical way to increase your sexual comfort. Feeling familiar and comfortable with your genitals can enhance sexual experiences. Many women find it empowering when they explore and learn about their bodies. You can do the *Vulva-Selfie Tour* as many times as you like. You can do it on your own or you can do it with someone that you trust. If you are not ready to take yourself on a *Vulva-Selfie Tour* that is absolutely fine. You can still learn a lot about your anatomy by reading about it.

However, if you're ready to dive down-under, then doing a regular *Vulva-Selfie Tour* is an excellent way for you to monitor any changes that can occur during the many years of your vulva ownership. Knowing what your *normal* looks like will help you to notice any changes in your vulval appearance that may require medical attention. *Vulva-Selfies* should not replace a regular genital or pelvic examination by your general practitioner. Your *Vulva-Selfie Tour* is a visual experience, as well as a tactile experience, where you can feel the texture of the different parts of vulva as you explore them.

Because our vulva is hidden away, many girls and women have never seen their own vulva. Here are some steps to easily find your way around your vulva. It is important to wash your hands before you begin touching your vulva and vagina. This is to avoid contaminating your vulva, especially your urethral opening with bacteria on your hands, which can lead to a UTI (urinary tract infection). The best time for your first *Vulva-Selfie Tour* is when you are between your menstrual cycles.

To get the tour started, follow these steps:

- You will need to get a hand-held mirror. Alternatively, you could use the camera on your mobile phone in selfie mode. You might find it easier to use a mirror with a stand or your phone with a holder so you can easily adjust the position and angle so you can see your genitals more clearly.

- It might also help to use lubricant as you go on your *Vulva-Selfie Tour* but it is not essential.

- You will need a torch or a bright lamp so you can directly illuminate your vulva and can see it more clearly. You can try aiming the torch at your genitals or in the mirror for better illumination.

- You can make a visual representation when exploring your clitoris (which reigns above and below the skin), grab a tape-measure or ruler or download a ruler app.

- It is important to find a comfortable space, that is private where you won't be disturbed. You can recline on a chair, sit up on your bed or sit on the floor – make sure your back is supported with pillows.

- Take your clothes off below the waist.

- Bend your knees, place your feet near your bottom and lean slightly backward and spread your knees apart so your genital area can be seen. You will be more comfortable on your *Vulva-Selfie Tour* if you relax your pelvic and stomach muscles.

- Make sure you have the *Your Amazing Vulva* and *Your Amazing Clitoris* diagrams – take a photo of them on your phone for easy reference and have them close by so you can identify the different parts of your vulva as you go.

It is important while on your *Vulva-Selfie Tour* to have a mindset of mindfulness, curiosity and wonderment as you start to explore yourself. As you are doing your *Vulva-Selfie Tour*, it is important to reflect on your genital image – and how diverse, like any other part of the human body, women's vulvas are in appearance. They, too, come in all shapes and sizes.

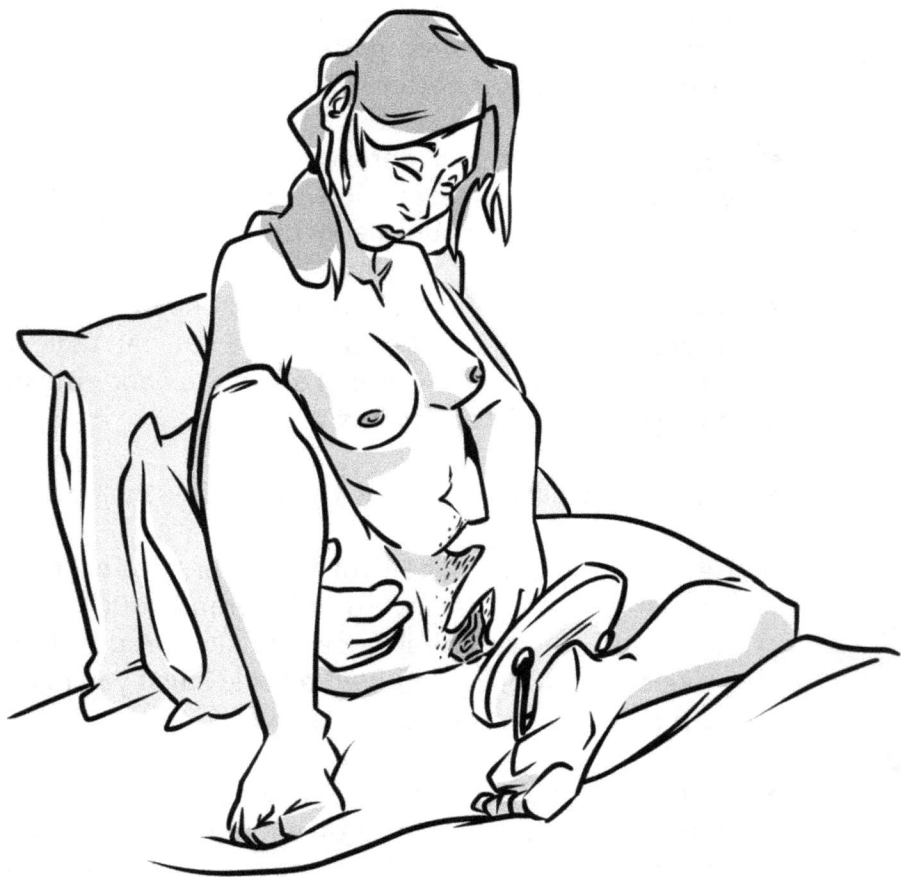

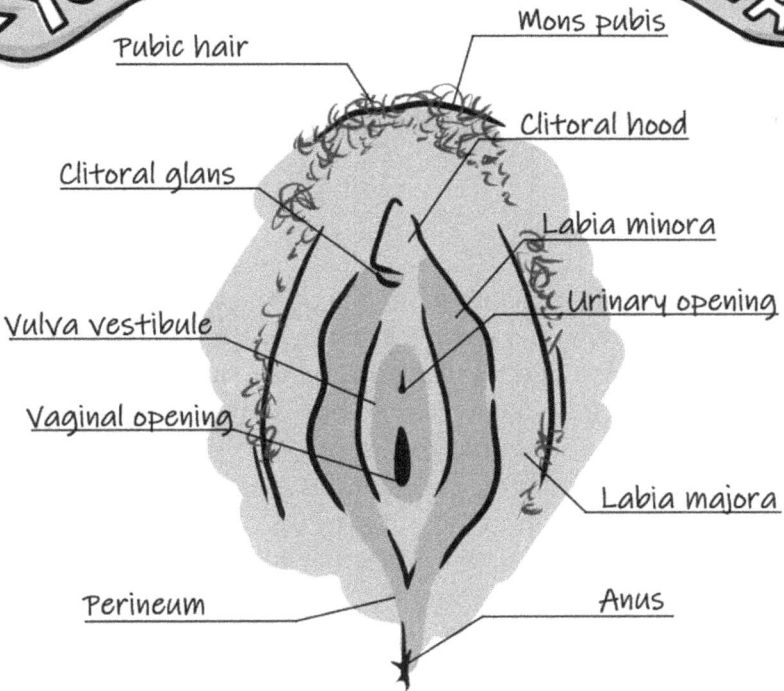

YOUR AMAZING VULVA

Pubic hair

Mons pubis

Clitoral hood

Clitoral glans

Labia minora

Urinary opening

Vulva vestibule

Vaginal opening

Labia majora

Perineum

Anus

Pubic Hair & Mons Pubis

Your Map of Tassie & Hairy Cushion Makes Sex Better

We start the *Vulva-Selfie Tour* from the outside area and then we will work our way between the folds of the labia majora. The first place we are going to stop at, is the pubic hair. Pubic hair, also known as *pubes*, covers the mons pubis and the outer edges of your labia majora. Your upholstery may even grow on your inner thighs and around your anus. The first wisps of pubic hair appear at puberty and are an early sign of development. At puberty, pubic hair is soft and darkish. Later your pubic hair will become longer, curly, thick and coarse. Some women's pubic hair may be straight while others' may be wavy. All variations and combinations of the texture, length, colour and distribution of pubic patches are normal. There is great variation in the growth pattern of pubic hair between women. Your pubic hair is the most obvious feature of your vulva, unless you practice pubic hair grooming, such as shaving, waxing or LASER hair removal. The pubic hair and/or the mons pubis are often the only part of women's genitalia you may have seen in sports changing rooms or when you have seen family members getting changed at home.

Why do I have pubic hair? Your pubic patch is a sign of adult female sexuality. It serves as a visual cue that signals your sexual maturity to those who see your pubic hair. It is suggested that the texture of your pubic hair is thicker and coarser than the hair on your head because it acts as a dry lubricant. During sexual activity, your hairy cushion acts as a buffer to lessen friction burns, skin abrasions and rashes. It is also suggested that pubic hair acts as a natural barrier and protects your genitals by preventing the spread or transmission of sexually transmitted infections (STIs). Going bare down there can increase the risk of you getting genital warts, chlamydia, gonorrhoea, syphilis or herpes. However, having pubic hair alone is not enough to protect you against STIs. The hairy barrier also protects your genitals from vulvar and vaginal irritation and infection. It also serves to protect your genitals from the cold and absorbs perspiration. Pubic hair may also play a role in sexual arousal – each one of your pubic hairs is attached to a nerve ending and when it is tugged at during sex, this causes traction and stimulates your touch receptors. Your pubic hair is truly a magic carpet! Just because many women remove some or all of their pubic hair does not mean that it shouldn't be there. If you choose to remove it, that is up to you, but there is nothing abnormal about having pubic hair.

Your mons pubis, also known as mons, is a pad of fatty tissue that covers your pubic bone The size of the mons pubis has many natural variations and all are normal. The primary purpose of your *mountain of Venus* is to provide cushioning. It protects your pelvic bone and other genital structures, from all the bumping and grinding that can occur during sexual intercourse.

MUFF MYTH: Your mons pubis secretes pheromones which are trapped by your pubic hair to attract sexual partners.

FANNY FACT: Scientists suggest the possibility that human secretions and odours do play a role in sexual attraction and selection, but the theory remains unproven.

LABIA MAJORA

YOUR OUTER GENITAL LIPS FORM A COVERING FOR THE OPENINGS BELOW

Where are my labia majora? Your labia majora or outer labia are where the pubic hair grows. Just like your mons pubis, the labia majora becomes covered by pubic hair after the onset of puberty. Your labia majora surround your *clitoral glans*, labia minora, vaginal opening, urethral opening and vulva vestibule. Your labia majora are the two hairy folds of skin that extend downward from your mons pubis and downward to your perineum. The appearance of the labia majora is different between women and can range in size, shape and colour – all variations in appearance are normal. The colour of the outside skin of women's labia majora is usually close to the colour of her overall skin colour. The pudendal cleft is also called the *cleft of Venus* and is the opening between the labia majora. It is located at the lower part of the mons pubis and separates the mons pubis into the labia majora.

Vulva-Selfie Tour – If you gently spread apart your labia majora at the pudendal cleft junction you will see or feel your labia minora. You can also see that your labia majora are protecting your vestibule. You will notice that the inside skin and mucus membrane of your labia majora may be pink or brownish, although there is considerable variation among women. The inside skin of the labia majora has a smooth, hairless surface and may feel moist when you touch it. You may notice on your *Vulva-Selfie Tour* that when you touch or apply a little pressure to your labia majora you experience a pleasurable sensation – this is because of the numerous nerve endings.

Why do I have labia majora? The labia majora are amazing because they contain and protect the more delicate parts of your vulva. When women are sexually aroused or having sexy thoughts their labia majora may feel tingly and warm. This is because the labia majora are sensitive and tighten up during sexual arousal. Also, during sexual arousal the labia majora spread apart and flatten to expose the clitoris.

On the surface of the skin of the labia majora are hair follicles, sweat glands and *sebaceous glands* called *sebum*. Sebum is an oily-like substance and has a protective role by waterproofing the labia majora and preventing urine, menstrual blood and bacteria from sticking to the surface. Sebum is that slippery feeling you have when sexually aroused which protects your vulva by absorbing friction during sexual intercourse. Just beneath the skin layer of the labia majora there is also a lot going on, with fatty tissue, ligaments, smooth muscle fibres, nerves, blood and lymphatic vessels.

MUFF MYTH: You should keep your labia majora, and the rest of your vulva and vagina, smelling fresh.

FANNY FACT: *V-odour* does not mean you have bad hygiene. Your vulva and vagina have a scent that is normal. Your vulva has many sweat glands – so when you are sweaty, your vulva will produce an odour. If you experience a strong odour, itchiness, unusual discharge or dryness it is important to speak to your doctor to have the symptoms checked out. The sooner you make an appointment to speak to your doctor the better, so you don't have to be worried. Doctors are used to talking to women about such concerns so there is no need to feel any embarrassment.

You can visit *The Vagina Museum* online for more muffbusters and fanny facts.

As your genitals are self-cleaning, using feminine hygiene products, particularly those that are perfumed or scented, can do more harm to the good bacteria that lives there. Washing everything away can alter the natural levels of your vaginal flora and lead to infections. For more information check out *Sexual Health and Family Planning Australia* for a clinic in your state or territory. You will be able to access excellent information on a number of conditions that can affect your vulva and vagina and things you can do to keep your vulva and vagina healthy.

Labia Minora

Your Delicate Inner Origami Folds

Where are my labia minora? The skin of your labia minora joins at the clitoral hood and extends past your urinary opening and vaginal opening. The inner genital lips surround the opening to your vagina. Your labia minora are dotted all over with sweat or oil glands called sebaceous glands. Your labia minora are also dotted with *Skene's glands* and *Bartholin's glands*, which produce mucus and other lubricants. Your inner lips are also made up of blood vessels and nerve endings. Prior to the onset of puberty, the labia minora are typically small and flat. During puberty, the labia minora gradually enlarge and grow to adult size. The labia minora can shrink and reduce in size after menopause.

Vulva-Selfie Tour – From majora to minora – if you gently spread apart your labia majora, you will see your labia minora. Your labia minora are the delicate, two hairless folds of skin that are within your labia majora. Your labia minora may appear darker in colour, than your labia majora. If you gently feel the skin of your labia minora, you will feel tiny bumps that might feel a little grainy to touch. These are the sebaceous glands.

The texture and appearance of the skin of the labia minora differ between women and can range from a smooth surface to a mildly wrinkled or corrugated surface of the outer or free edge. You will notice that your inner labia will feel warmer and moister than your labia majora. This is where the normal skin secretions from neighbouring areas of your vulva and vagina accumulate. This lubrication protects your vulva against irritation from the different structures rubbing against one another. Clever vulva!

The labia minora are a very important part of the sexual response. When you are not aroused or sexually stimulated, the labia minora cover the vaginal and urethral openings. When you are aroused and in a sexually stimulating situation, the labia minora become more open.

The labia minora are composed mainly of elastic fibres and blood vessels and are very rich in sensory nerve endings and receptors. This arrangement within the labia minora forms erectile tissue. The edges of the labia minora are also rich in sensory nerve endings and are also involved in the process of engorgement during sexual arousal. With sexual arousal, the labia minora will swell to become bigger and wider as they become engorged with blood. Their dimensions can double or triple in size at peak arousal. Your labia minora become plump little pillows and move away from your vaginal opening (*introitus*) to make way for sexual penetration. How amazing is that! Post-arousal you can expect your labia minora to return to their former appearance in a short period of time.

The labia minora are there for your sexual pleasure. Many women feel that their labia minora are second only to their clitoris for sexual sensation and sexual sensitivity. Oodles of women also feel that they experience more sexual pleasure and sensation through their clitoris and labia minora – more so than their vagina.

Who knew that such a small part of your amazing body could do so much and be so important to your sexual functioning and arousal? Your labia minora are unique – they will vary significantly from the labia minora of other girls and women in shape, size, symmetry and skin colouration.

Innie wings and outie wings. The shape, size and symmetry of your labia minora are highly individualised and range from short to long. One labium (singular of labia) can be smaller than the other labium or they can both be of similar size. Your little wings might not look the same on each side – one wing might be longer or wider than the other wing. One wing might be fatter or thinner than the other wing. They can be thin, thick or bumpy too.

The labia minora can protrude between the labia majora in some women, but in others, the labia minora can be covered by the labia majora. The labia minora can change in size – *innies* may become more *outies* when you have sexy thoughts or are feeling horny.

Many shades of you. The colour of your labia minora is highly individualised and ranges from different shades of pink to different shades of brown and can be purplish in colour. The labia minora may be a different skin colour than the area surrounding it. The colour of your labia minora is unique and these colours varies from individual to individual. The labia minora can change in colour – they become darker during sexual arousal. With sexual arousal the labia minora will change colour as they become engorged with blood. The labia minora may also darken during pregnancy.

Colour changes that occur to my labia minora and why? The edges of women's labia minora tend to darken in colour around the time of adolescence or during pregnancy. Adolescence and pregnancy are reproductive milestones and colour changes naturally occur at these times due to increases in women's hormone levels. It is normal and natural for the edge of women's labia minora to appear darker than the rest of their labia minora skin colour.

Labia minora and vulvovaginal health. The labia minora also play an important role in maintaining vulvovaginal health. Just like the labia majora – your labia minora, with their two folds of skin, act as a barrier against infection and external irritants. The labia minora enclose and protect the urethral opening and inner parts of the vagina from infection. The labia minora also play a significant role in directing the urine stream while you wee. If you didn't have your little wings, your wee would spray everywhere!

The labia minora and labia majora protect the urethral opening and the vaginal opening. When you are in a sexually unstimulated situation, your labia minora cover your vaginal and urethral openings. The labia minora act like a little gate that covers the entrance of your vagina called the *introitus*. When you are in a sexually stimulating situation (getting turned-on), your labia minora become more open and your urethra shows changes in blood flow as well. The labia minora also protects the clitoral glans. The upper layer of the labia minora passes above the clitoris then joins to form a fold called the clitoral hood.

TAKE HOME MESSAGE Your labia minora are unique. There is no *normal* appearance – how your labia minora appears is *your normal*. Have a look online at *The Labia Library* to get a sense of how varied the overall appearance of women's vulvas can be.

MUFF MYTH: If you have lots of penetrative sex your labia minora will get longer.

FANNY FACT: The shape and size of your labia minora is in no way affected by the amount of penetrative sex you have. Labia minora growth and development is a part of puberty. Your labia minora may change in appearance throughout the lifespan (puberty, pregnancy and menopause).

Your Clitoris Reigns Above & Below Your Body

The clitoris is pure in purpose.
It is the only organ in the body designed purely for pleasure.
– Eve Ensler

So far on your *Vulva-Selfie Tour* you have gotten to know the *Amazing Four*: pubic hair, mons pubis, labia majora and labia minora. They are a force to be reckoned with, act as protectors and also have their role to play in female sexuality. Now let's have a look at the part of our genital anatomy that most of us refer to as the clitoris. Some women call their clitoris the *clit*. They are referring to that little nub that we can see and feel. Its anatomical name is the *clitoral glans* or *glans clitoris and* it is responsible for bringing us delicious sexual pleasure and sensation.

Research is changing the way we think about female sexuality. Our amazing clitoris was not accurately anatomically mapped and described until 1998 by a team of Australian urological surgeons led by Australia's first female urologist surgeon,

Professor Helen O'Connell. Go Aussies! Can you believe it – our clitoris had been left in the dark and neglected by medical science and research for so long? Let's now find out more about this wondrous sexual organ.

It may come as a very pleasant surprise to you to learn that there is much more to the clitoris than meets the eye and it is made up of external and internal parts. The clitoris is described as a multi-planar structure – this means that it has many structures or components. These clitoral components are complimentary and symbiotic. The structures make up a unique and complex three-dimensional arrangement as illustrated in the *Your Amazing Clitoris* diagram. Also check out the superimposed diagram of *Your Amazing Clitoris and Vulva*. By knowing and owning all the information you can about your clitoris it will help build your sexual self-esteem and confidence. It's your body after all and what you learn here can help you to educate your sexual partner too.

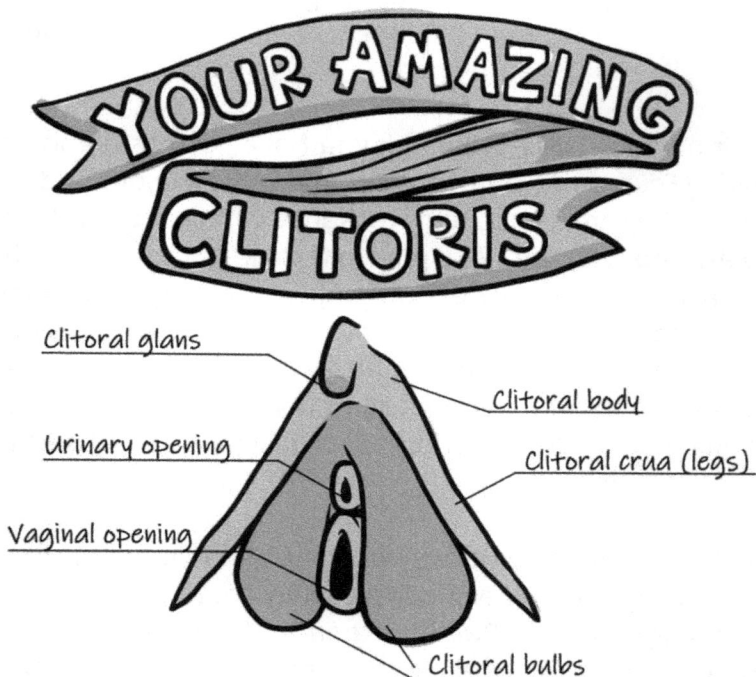

YOUR AMAZING CLITORIS

Clitoral glans
Clitoral body
Urinary opening
Clitoral crua (legs)
Vaginal opening
Clitoral bulbs

ON THE SURFACE: WOMEN'S SEXUAL AROUSAL REIGNS HERE

Vulva-Selfie Tour – If you gently spread apart your labia majora and look just above your urethral opening, you will see where two folds of your labia minora join up. It is here you will see a small fold of skin – you have found your clitoral hood. The appearance of clitoral hoods can vary in size and in the degree of coverage from woman to woman. All variations in the appearance of clitoral hoods are normal.

Gently wiggle the clitoral hood with your fingertips, you can also gently press down if you like and you will feel a rounded elevation. This little bump is your clitoris glans and is about 2 to 3 centimetres long with a similar diameter. For some women, it is easier to see when they spread apart their vulva and can see it sitting snugly beneath their clitoral hood. Some women notice that their clitoral hood retracts easily. Other women might find that it does not pull back – either way is perfectly normal.

Now, it is time to have a further peek or feel under the hood of your clitoral glans. If you are able to, gently pull apart the skin and you will see more clearly this pea-sized nub-like structure which is often referred to as a *magic button*. Your magic button requires a gentle, soft touch – simply pressing it like it is an on/off light switch can be very uncomfortable. I recommend you make your enquiry using gentle pressure and motions.

Your clitoral glans is very small, but it has a huge personality. It is an amazing part of your vulva. For starters, your clitoral glans contains a very high concentration of nerve endings. It has 8,000 nerve endings, which is twice as many found in the *penis*! The clitoris is the female equivalent of the penis. The penis has reproductive, sexual and urinary functions, whereas the clitoris has only one function in female sexuality and that is sexual pleasure. All of these nerve endings make the clitoris extremely sensitive to touch. The sole purpose of these thousands and thousands of nerve endings is for creating sexual pleasure and orgasm. If you touch your clitoral glans directly (*ouch!*) it can feel less pleasurable than touching your clitoral glans through your clitoral hood (*woo-hoo!*). The clitoral hood is there to protect this highly sensitive and highly erotic part of your body.

If you gently rub through your clitoral hood, you will be able to feel the clitoral body underneath the skin. The clitoral body is surrounded by fibroelastic tissue. You may also be able to see the shape or the outline of the clitoral body under your skin and it may feel like a little tube and firm to the touch. The clitoral glans surrounds the body of the clitoris is partly visible and then disappears below the surface of the vulva. The shape of the clitoral body varies in size and shape among women and comes in many combinations. For instance, some might be long and thin or short and thick – all combinations are considered to be normal. The appearance of the clitoral hood and clitoral glans also differ between women with a wide variation in size, shape, colour and texture.

The clitoral glans has a very small proportion of erectile tissue compared to its subterranean parts. The major role of the clitoral glans is for sensation and during sexual arousal and stimulation, can become swollen but not erect or rigid. Some women report that one side of their clitoral glans feels more sensitive compared to the other side.

SUBTERRANEAN PARTS:
A WOMEN'S ERECTION
HAPPENS INSIDE HER BODY

Many people think the clitoral glans is the whole of the clitoris, but the clitoral glans is like a little cap and is quite *clit-erally* the tip of the iceberg. Around ninety percent of your clitoral anatomy happens beneath the surface of your vulva. These components contain erectile tissue that swell and become erect when you get turned on. Most of your erection happens under your vulval skin which can't be seen but you can feel parts of the swelling through the skin. There is variation in the size and shape of women's subterranean clitoral anatomy and all expressions are normal.

Under your public bone and vulvar skin are the deeper structures of your clitoris that consist of the *body* (*corpora*), *root*, *paired crura* and *clitoral bulbs*. The shape of your clitoris in its 3D glory has been described as looking like a boomerang or a plump wishbone. For me, the shape of the clitoris in its entirety looks like a space-age penguin.

Vulva-Selfie Tour – As the next part of your *Vulva-Selfie Tour* is subterranean you can use your ruler, tape measure or ruler app along with *Your Amazing Clitoris* diagram. These travel tools will give you a visual reference of the proportions of your hidden clitoral empire.

Your clitoral body peeps above the surface of your vulval skin – it is also hidden below. Typically, the body of the clitoris is between 1 to 2 centimetres wide – as wide as the first joint of your thumb. It is possible to feel your clitoral body by placing your finger where your labia minora meets, then place your thumb above the clitoral hood and give a gentle roll and a little squeeze. The clitoral body sort of feels like a rubber band and may move easily when you apply a little pressure. Some women find it easier to locate when they are sexually aroused. The clitoral body is made up of erectile tissue called *corpora cavernosa* – which are expandable sponge-like tissue that play a very important role in women's sexual arousal. When you are sexually aroused the little pockets of space or little caves, within the corpus cavernosa fill up with blood and become erect. In this erotic state your clitoral body will become raised and feel firm to the touch.

The clitoral body is between 2 to 4 centimetres long (about as long as the tip of your thumb to the first joint) and fan out into two legs called the *clitoral crura*. The clitoral crura are narrower than the clitoral body and are between 5 to 9 centimetres long (about as long your index finger). The clitoral crura lie either side of your urethral and vaginal openings. They are also made up of the same erectile tissue as the clitoral body. When you are sexually aroused, the clitoral crura engorge with blood and become erect.

The clitoral bulbs look like two teardrop or eggplant shapes and are between 3 to 7 centimetres long and are also made up of erectile tissue called *corpus spongiosum*. They fill the space between the clitoral crura. During sexual arousal when pleasure is induced, they become more sensitive and expand in size – this is what also creates your erection. The clitoral bulbs drape over the upper side of your urethra and either side of your vaginal wall. During vaginal penetration, you may feel sexual pleasure due to the clitoral bulbs sitting on either side of your vagina and urethra. It has been suggested that when your bulbs are engorged, this aids in vaginal penetration by making the anterior walls of the vagina rigid.

The *clitoral root* forms the connection with your clitoral body, clitoral crura and clitoral bulbs. The convergence of these clitoral erectile bodies is very important in sexual sensation. The clitoral root lies behind your urethral opening. Its location is very close to the surface and can be stimulated directly when the area is touched. Women have erections too! The pars intermedia is also a very important anatomical area of the clitoris. The pars intermedia consists of channels, or a conduit of blood vessels, that unite all the clitoral parts and lie just beneath the skin.

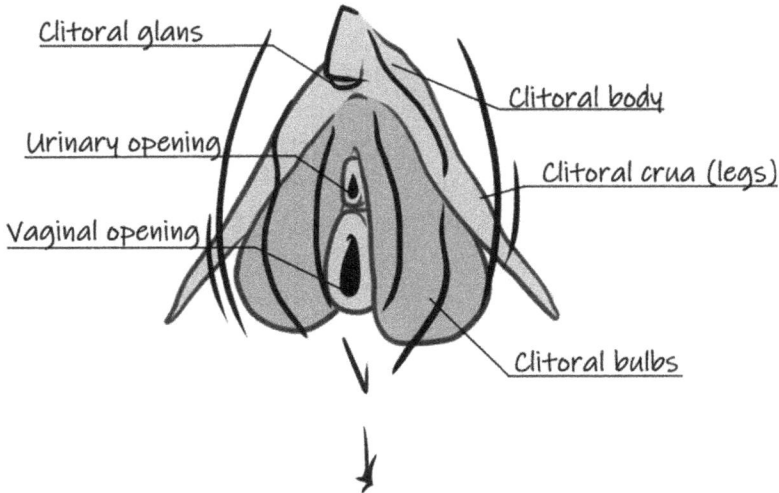

YOUR AMAZING VULVA + CLITORIS

Clitoral glans

Urinary opening

Vaginal opening

Clitoral body

Clitoral crua (legs)

Clitoral bulbs

Perfect Harmony

Your Body and Brain Create Your Female Orgasm

These *fab four* subterranean erectile structures of your clitoris, along with their above terrain sisters, all work in perfect harmony for your sexual pleasure and female orgasm.

The sequence of events that lead to female orgasm goes something like this. When the sensory nerve fibres of the clitoris glans are stimulated this causes sexual pleasure and in turn sends sensory information or chemical messages to the brain. The chemical messages the brain receives (*OMG, here is sexual pleasure!*) activate another set of chemical messages (*let's get this party started!*), that then causes the spongy erectile tissues in the clitoris to expand and *voila*, erection of the clitoris occurs. This pressure build-up makes the clitoral glans swell and it retracts into the clitoral hood. Meanwhile, the labia minora become erect, the vagina becomes lubricated, then your pelvic area will experience waves of muscle contractions and you will have an orgasm. *Wow!*

Of course, the female sexual response is more complex than this description. Researchers with new technology and methodology are still making new discoveries about how our genitals and our brains work in harmony to create sexual pleasure.

MUFF BUSTER TIME

THE HOLLYWOOD FEMALE ORGASM SCRIPT: THE GREAT CLITORAL ORGASM COVERUP

We live in a fantasy world, a world of illusion.
The great task in life is to find reality.

– Iris Murdoch

Depictions of women having mind-blowing orgasms every time they have sex in films and TV shows are Hollywood sex, not real-life sex. Essentially, the industry is dominated by men who write, direct and produce films and TV shows. *The Hollywood Female Orgasm Script* is simple and time-limited. Actors are directed and paid to *act out* sex in a fast and furious fashion. The essential ingredient for film and TV producers is to portray women having screaming orgasms every time. The female actor is directed to climax very quickly and often at the male actor's first touch or their first forceful pelvic thrust. The Hollywood orgasm script all occurs in under a minute! Here is the script – I think you will recognise it as the format itself is standard to the genre:

Action – Start of scene: Man and woman have an urgent and furious open mouth gnashing of teeth to simulate passionate kissing (1–10 seconds). Woman is hoisted up and slammed against a wall or thrown down on the bed for a bit of missionary (1–10 seconds). Woman has an eye-rolling screaming orgasm soon after man squirms around on her (1–10 seconds). Woman and man roll around and fall off one another (1–10 seconds). Phone rings and woman or man answers the phone (1–10 seconds). **Cut – End of scene.**

Hollywood sex is fake sex – where there is no consent, no safe-sex discussion, no foreplay, no time for arousal, no feedback, no emotion, no relationship and no seduction. It is based on what producers in Hollywood want the female orgasm to be. The industry is not going to change as these people hold dear the viewpoint that sensational sex sells. Real-life sex does not make for good viewing, nor the ratings. Everyday sex is vanilla sex and is considered too bland and boring – not good for the bank balance of the movie moguls and shareholders. Many of us know that Hollywood sex is not realistic nor an accurate portrayal of how women actually orgasm. Hollywood has oversimplified the female orgasm.

However, the images we see on the screens are incredibly powerful and we can easily and unconsciously internalise this Hollywood stereotype. Our expectations of the sex that is depicted by Hollywood can transfer into our romantic lives. The very big problem is that this misinformation is transferred into our bedrooms. This can cause distress for individuals and couples. In my private practice, I have met many couples whose relationships are in trouble when either one or both of them has subscribed to the Hollywood myth of male and female sexuality. That is, where men are portrayed to be wanting sex all the time and women are always available for sex and have frenzied screaming orgasms. Hollywood sex and pornography give us all (both men and women) the misbelief that there is only one kind of orgasm and that is the vaginal orgasm.

Often, women would present to my rooms for counselling on how to have an orgasm. More often than not, they would be there on their own – full of self-blame, shame and embarrassment. They would tell me that their male sexual partner told them that something is wrong with them. The male partner believed that if their wife or girlfriend could not have an orgasm during penile-vaginal sex, it is the woman who has the problem. With no thanks to Hollywood, pornography, lack of sex education or dud lovers, for many women their orgasm will remain elusive. The antidote is to challenge these erroneous portrayals of female sexuality by raising our awareness and knowledge about female sexuality. That is, to not only educate ourselves but our sexual partners that the clitoris is how most women experience orgasms and not the vagina.

Women are looking for a cure to a problem that doesn't exist. Men are not the experts when it comes to female sexuality and especially female orgasm. I found in my private practice that in many instances, the male partner was not very well informed about women's sexuality. The best outcomes were when couples worked together. Those who challenged their misbeliefs and misperceptions of Hollywood scripted sex were able to re-build their relationship and increase their confidence in the bedroom.

Fanny Fact Time

The Female Orgasm is Borne from the Clitoris

This fanny fact is about dispelling the vaginal orgasm myth and how before Hollywood, there was psychoanalyst Sigmund Freud who in 1905 invented the term *vaginal orgasm*. Freud is recognised for starting the vaginal orgasm myth. His theory is considered by many researchers and health professionals as arrogant, and even dangerous to women's sexual health. This misbelief has caused women tremendous problems and has haunted female sexuality ever since. Today, it is generally considered among the medical and academic communities, that the clitoris is the only sex organ best equipped for the female orgasm. The vagina has very low sensitivity and many women do not have orgasms during sexual intercourse or penetrative sexual activity alone. There are women who report they have vaginal orgasms and this in all likelihood is caused by the surrounding erectile tissue of the clitoris.

Female sexual pleasure or sexual arousal originates in many parts of the body, generally in the vulva, and more specifically in the clitoris for sexual climax. It is the pumping or thrusting action that occurs during vaginal intercourse that causes the necessary friction and the vagina provides the best lubrication (if the woman is aroused enough) that men require to reach their orgasm. Men have their own unique way to climax which is very, very different to the unique way in which women climax. The function of the clitoris is for our sexual pleasure and for the female orgasm. The vagina is a multitasker – it is there for menstruation, allows the penis to enter, holds semen and is a passage for a baby to be born. The vagina is also an erotic centre, but not the centre for orgasms. For best orgasmic results, many women find that stimulating their clitoral glans during sexual intercourse will increase their sexual pleasure and the likelihood of having a more intense orgasm.

By talking specifically to your partner about what makes sex more enjoyable and pleasurable for you, you just might find that you won't feel as if you have to fake your orgasms anymore! Many of the women I have seen are too embarrassed to talk about sex with their partner in such an explicit way. The more comfortable you and your partner are with sexual communication, the more pleasurable the sexual experience will be for you both. For a starting point I recommend reading *Good Loving, Great Sex* by Dr Rosie King, *When Your Sex Drives Don't Match* by Dr Sandra Pertot and *The Elusive Orgasm* by Dr Vivienne Cass – these are excellent resources by Australian female authors. You will learn that no two orgasms are alike and that libidos come in all shapes and sizes too.

Sexual difficulties are a couple's issue, not an individual issue. Ideally, the couple both need to be reading and talking through issues together. By working through the exercises together this helps the couple to have a greater appreciation of how to have a more satisfying sex life. Engaging with the reading and doing the exercises outlined in the afore-mentioned books, helps the couple become better sexual communicators. If your partner is not wanting to read any of the resources, so be it – not ideal but absolutely fine. You can become your own sex therapist – the new information you have absorbed will enable you to be more comfortable with your own sexuality. Another benefit that women find is that they become more comfortable about intimacy. For other women they realise that there was absolutely nothing wrong with them to begin with – they just didn't have the appropriate knowledge or know-how.

THE HYMEN (VAGINAL CORONA)

MYTHS & REALITIES REVEALED

*The mythical status of the hymen
has caused far too much harm for far too long.*
**– The Swedish Association for
Sexuality Education**

The hymen/vaginal corona. To help dispel the many myths surrounding the hymen, *The Swedish Association for Sexuality Education*, a Swedish sexual rights group renamed the hymen to be called the *vaginal corona*. However, for most of us, the word *hymen* is a more familiar term. The hymen/vaginal corona has no known biological function. One theory suggests that it is a remnant of foetal development and evolved to work as a barrier to prevent vaginal infections.

Where is my hymen/vaginal corona? Myths about the hymen/vaginal corona may have arisen from the common misunderstanding that the hymen/vaginal corona is a brittle membrane that covers the vaginal opening. In fact, the membrane lies within 0.5 to 2 centimetres of the vaginal opening. If you gently separate your labia minora and look into your vaginal opening, you may or may not be able to see your hymen/vaginal corona, or you might notice some remnants. The hymen/vaginal corona is made up of elastic mucous tissue folds, which may cover all or part of the vaginal opening. Your hymen/vaginal corona can disappear for all sorts of reasons. For a very small proportion of women, their hymen/vaginal corona has been absent since birth. Simply looking to see if a woman has a hymen/vaginal corona says absolutely nothing about whether they have had sexual intercourse. As such, the presence of the hymen/vaginal corona is an inappropriate measure of women's virginity, just as you can't prove whether or not a man is a virgin by looking at his penis or testicles.

It is a myth that the hymen/vaginal corona ruptures and bleeds the first time a woman has sexual intercourse. Many women report no bleeding at their first intercourse. The hymen/vaginal corona can break or stretch during non-sexual activity, including surgical procedures such as speculum examinations, tampon insertion, masturbation or any form of vaginal penetration. It is a common assumption that vigorous exercise or sporting activities may also rupture the hymen/vaginal corona. Engaging in vigorous sporting activities such as gymnastics or horseback riding does not cause hymenal/vaginal coronal changes.

In the same way that every woman's vulva is different, every woman's hymen/vaginal corona is different too. The hymen/vaginal corona can naturally vary a lot in appearance and comes in different colours and shapes. The hymen/vaginal corona is a rim of tissue at the vaginal opening and may appear transparent, red, purple, pink or whitish and the tissue may either be thick or thin. It can be a donut or a half-moon shape, fringed, have several holes or lobes, or it can be absent altogether. For some women their membrane is very elastic and stretchy and can sustain the penetration of a finger, tampon or penis, etcetera, without making it completely disappear. There is no standardisation of what constitutes an intact hymen/vaginal corona. All anatomical variants in the appearance of the hymen/vaginal corona are normal. Virginity is not a medical condition and there is no medical definition of virginity based on hymenal/vaginal coronal appearance.

THE G-SPOT

MYTHS & REALITIES REVEALED

The G-spot is in the ears and anyone who goofs around looking for it any further down is wasting his time and ours.

– Isabel Allende

Has anyone seen the G-spot? The G-spot is also called the *Gräfenberg spot* after the German gynaecologist Ernst Gräfenberg who in 1950 noted a sensitive area along the anterior of the vaginal wall. However, the existence of this erogenous zone has never been found. The G-spot is not a distinct anatomical structure. Despite that no distinct anatomical structure has been found by researchers, many women, the media and health professionals continue to believe in its mystical existence.

Do vaginal orgasms exist? The mystical status of the G-spot has caused far too much orgasm angst for a long time. Many women believe that this erotic zone causes vaginal orgasms. Women report that a vaginal orgasm is more intense than the orgasm they experience when their clitoral glans is stimulated. There is an area about one third of the way up from the vaginal opening on the front wall (your belly-button side) of your vagina and when this area is stimulated, some women experience intense sexual pleasure and experience a vaginal orgasm(s). The pleasure that some women feel when this area is stimulated during sexual arousal is probably explained by the highly sensitive clitoris and not by an area on the vaginal wall. It is suggested that the lower third of the anterior wall of the vagina is sensitive and the movement of this area by a finger, penis or sex toy causes pressure on the clitoris. Just below the skin of this area of the vaginal wall are the clitoral bulbs. Some women will have more extensive clitoral tissues and nerves than others and therefore women's experience of an orgasm will be varied. So, because of the clitoral bulb's proximity to the vaginal wall, it is considered to be a clitoral orgasm and not a vaginal orgasm. Mystery solved! There is only one type of orgasm achieved through vaginal penetration – an inner clitoral one. Well, not quite – the mystery has not been completely solved. Researchers are only beginning to map and describe this amazing part of women's genital anatomy and its role in the female sexual response.

Vulva-Selfie Tour - If you want to find your sensitive area, it is best to do so when you are very turned on – place your finger just inside your vagina (about 5 to 8 centimetres) and press up towards your pubic bone in a come-hither motion. You might find it easier to explore your G-spot by sitting with your knees up. Every woman is different in their orgasmic experience. Some women don't find this area to be very sensitive at all when they are sexually excited. This is completely normal as everyone's bodies, including their clitoral anatomy are different. For some women they are not bothered if they don't orgasm during sex. However, other women who are not able to orgasm during any sort of sexual activity experience a great deal of concern. Orgasms can be elusive and there are many reasons why women don't orgasm. *The Elusive Orgasm* by Dr Vivienne Cass, an Australian clinical psychologist, is an excellent resource for women who want to find out why they can't orgasm and learn how to get there.

Vulva Vestibule, Urethral & Vaginal Openings

Your Entrances & Exits

The vulva vestibule is the area between your labia minora. You will notice a smooth surface that begins just below your clitoral glans. The *vulva vestibule* is the entrance way to your urethral and vaginal openings. Your vulva vestibule can be varying in colour from shades of pink, red and brown. The vascular tissue of the vulva vestibule engorges during sexual arousal.

The urethral opening is positioned above the vaginal opening and can be seen from the outside. The opening is tiny and hard to see or feel. It is not one of the female's sex organs – the *urethral opening* is part of the urinary tract system. It is a tube that allows urine (liquid waste from the food and drink you have consumed) to travel from your bladder and leave your body through the urethral opening. Your urethral opening is between the labia minora and resides below your clitoris and above your vaginal opening. If you are having a look at your genitals with your mirror and torch, when you see your vaginal opening, look up a little bit and you will see that your urethral opening is positioned between your vaginal opening and below your clitoris glans. It has been suggested that during sexual arousal when the clitoris is erect, it closes the urethral opening which prevents bacteria from travelling up to the bladder and causing infections.

The vaginal opening is also called the *introitus* and can also be seen from the outside. It is below your urethral opening and allows the passage of a baby and the entry of penis, finger or tampon. The vagina is also known as the birth canal and is located inside your body. The vulva protects the vaginal opening with its double door – the labia majora and the labia minora. Use your fingers to spread apart the labia minora and you should be able to see the reddish or pinkish walls of the vagina. The walls of the vagina have small folds or ridges known as rugae. Check out your vaginal discharge – a normal discharge is clear to cloudy white and smells slightly acidic like vinegar. The discharge may be thick or thin and changes throughout the menstrual cycle.

Perineum and Anus

Your Down Below of Your Down Below

Vulva-Selfie Tour – The second-to-last stop on your *Vulva-Selfie Tour* is your *perineum*. The perineum is the area of skin between your vaginal opening and anal opening. It lies where your labia majora ends and plays a very important function in stretching during childbirth. The final stop on the *Vulva-Selfie Tour* is the anus which is also called your anal opening. This exit allows the passing of poo and farts. No tour of your vulva would be complete without mentioning these two down-under structures.

Congratulations, Vulva Image Warrior! This is the end of the *Vulva-Selfie Tour*. Next up on your *Vulva Image Warrior* journey is to explore the different reasons why some women develop genital image troubles and anxieties.

V-SECTION TWO

Vulnerable Vulvas
Why Do Genital Anxieties Exist?

The increasingly specific and visible vulval ideal is that of a clean slit.

– Lindy McDougall

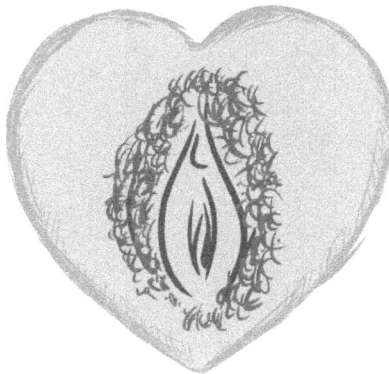

FAKE NEWS = POOR GENITAL IMAGE

Genital image research has found more women are becoming concerned about the appearance and function of their genitalia. In Australia, health professionals and researchers have reported a dramatic increase in the demand for female genital cosmetic surgery. This trend has also been observed in other Western countries, including the United States, Europe and the United Kingdom. The emergence of female genital cosmetic surgery has been attributed to sociocultural changes. This section will explore the external pressures from society that are creating internal turmoil for women and girls and the development of poor genital image. This section will also explore how these pressures are contributing to the increased popularity of female genital cosmetic surgery. Before you read on, I would like to redirect you to the YouTube video: *Dr Vajayjay's! Privatize Those Privates!* Dr Vajayjay explores how misinformation about vulval normalcy is perpetrated and disseminated in our culture. This video was created by *The New View Campaign*, a grassroots feminist activist group.

Hypersexualised Society

We all live in a hypersexualised society where there is increased visibility of the vulva with a focus on the groin. The increased popularity of female genital cosmetic surgery may be a product of living in a culture in which women's bodies, including their genitalia, are sexually objectified. We see highly sexualised images of women everywhere: pornography, magazines, social media, video games, music videos, performance art, billboards, television, merchandising, makeup and clothing advertisements. Sexual objectification leads women to internalise idealised sexualised body types. Living in a hypersexualised society places society's gaze on female genitalia. This may prompt some women to make negative comparisons between their own genitalia and the idealised images they see in the media. Women are getting cues that their vulvas are abnormal due to the failure of the media to acknowledge vulva diversity.

Ideal Genital Image

For decades, Western women have been trying to achieve the *ideal* body image and cosmetic surgery has been a way of achieving this. Women may have cosmetic surgery for aesthetic reasons, for example, to enlarge their breasts or flatten their stomach. This is seen as a normalised practical solution to achieve a perfect and desirable body. Women who are unhappy about the appearance and/or functionality of their genitals may also seek out cosmetic surgery to alter the appearance of their genitalia. These so-called *cosmetic* surgeries are not medically indicated and are potentially a serious health risk to women. *Designer vagina* surgeries are offered and marketed by clinics with claims of increasing sexual satisfaction or improving the appearance of the genitalia. The increase in female genital cosmetic surgery indicates that women are confused between what is idealised and what is normal genital appearance. The increase in women wanting to seek out surgery reflects a narrow cultural definition of what is normal and *desirable* genital appearance.

Altered Images

Understanding the Influence of Unrealistic Body & Genital Images

We live in a world where it is standard for the media to digitally alter body images. We know that many of these images are unrealistic, and even impossible, but they become deeply embedded in our self-perception in spite of this.

You don't have to be a graphic designer with the latest photo editing software to change a model's appearance. Manipulating and enhancing your own image can be easily achieved by accessing apps that retouch your own image. Low-cost apps and easy to use technology are readily available to get *Insta-ready*. You can click, choose, push, press or select to erase any blemishes, whiten your teeth, brighten your eyes and smooth away wrinkles. You can even make your limbs look longer, your breasts look bigger and slim down your waist, thighs and arms.

Altered images of women's genitalia are also standard in many women's magazines and softcore pornography. The result being every skerrick of pubic hair is airbrushed away, the mons pubis is flattened, the colour of the vulva is uniform and the labia minora are invisible.

This digital shapeshifting is known in the softcore pornography industry as keeping images of full-frontal nude female genitalia *neat and tidy*. The industry is only permitted to show a *clean slit*. Visible labia minora are considered too rude to be shown to the general public according to the Australian Classification system. It is possible that some women and men will be influenced by these *make-over fake-overs* which may lead them to develop unrealistic genital beauty aspirations and desires of their own.

To increase women's awareness of female genital diversity it is vitally important to increase your media literacy. An excellent resource is the YouTube video *The Labiaplasty Fad?* which addresses Australian censorship law and the labia minora. It will enlighten you on the disturbing process of digital alteration of female genitalia in the media and how these images make the real *unreal*. It clearly demonstrates to both women and men a narrow representation of women's genitals presented in the media – that is, allowing only one version of women's genital type to be deemed acceptable.

Porn Harms Kids

In 2016 at the *Pornography and Harm to Children and Young People Symposium: Porn Harm Kids* conference at the University of New South Wales in Sydney, I met Gladys (not her real name), who was in her late forties. Gladys worked in the education sector and was interested in learning more about the perceived harm being done to children and teens through early sexualisation and internet pornography exposure. She told me how pornography had shaped her own genital image. She recalled how as a teenager she was very curious about her father's softcore porn magazine collection that he had hidden in the back shed. She felt her genitals did not look like the images she had seen in her father's cache of *Penthouse*, *Picture* and *People* magazines. Gladys stated that she was extremely self-conscious about the appearance of her vulva, telling me she had '*too much chicken-skin*', referring to her labia minora. She was too self-conscious about her genital appearance to have a boyfriend for fear of rejection. In her early twenties, Gladys consulted two plastic surgeons for their opinion about having her labia minora reduced. Despite both plastic surgeons telling Gladys her labia minora were of normal appearance she still wanted to have her labia minora altered. Gladys recalled that at the time she didn't hesitate about her decision to have cosmetic surgery. Post-surgery she felt confident and sexy about herself and started to have boyfriends. In more recent years she had been reflecting on the effects of looking at softcore pornography and how it had shaped her sexual self-esteem. We both discussed and wondered what would have happened if Gladys had had the information available to her as a teen about genital image diversity and the way in which women's body and genital images are digitally altered in the media. Would the outcome be the same? Gladys commented if she were equipped with such knowledge as a teenager, she probably would not have worried about the appearance of her genitals and therefore would not have undergone cosmetic surgery.

Kids are viewing pornography younger than ever before. If you are wanting information on how to have tricky conversations and build porn-resilient kids, please check out *youthwellbeingproject.com.au* and *collectiveshout.org*

What's in a Name?

Growing up, we have learnt that the vulva and vagina have different names from those our mothers taught us and many of these terms are derogatory. Often, when women are talking about female genitals, they use different words in different situations. I used to call my vulva the *vagina* as that was the term my mother taught me as a child. As a teenager and in my twenties and beyond, among my friends, we would refer to our privates as *down-under, dick, pussy, box, minge, front bottom, map of Tassie, fanny, clit, vag, gina* and *lab.* I also recall we used the term *chicken skin* when referring to the grainy or pebbly texture and bumpy appearance of our labia minora. What we call our genitals and their different parts to the general practitioner or gynaecologist may be different from the name we use with our friends or lovers.

Our hidden down-under – our vulva and vagina – creates anxiety for many women. Education about naming the parts of our genitals will help stop genital image anxieties and engender empowerment. We live in a culture that considers these parts of the women's anatomy a mystery, even taboo. It is vital that our unmentionables become mentionable and be called by their correct names. This is a deeply personal issue for many and taboo for some. Viewing female genitalia as taboo is surprising, as despite living in a culture that publicly debates issues regarding sex and sexuality, the vulva and vagina continue to generate anxiety.

Taboo subjects tend to invite the use of euphemisms and slang terms. Many women refer to their female genitals by using terms such as *bits, down below, front bottom* or *fanny*. The use of euphemisms and slang terms are problematic as they strengthen the view that female genitalia are both taboo and offensive.

Many women regard their genitalia as something to be avoided in conversation at all costs, and as too difficult, shameful or embarrassing to talk about freely. Some women are very uncomfortable discussing their vulva and vagina-related issues with a healthcare professional. Similarly, some health professionals also have difficulty using the word vagina or even another word that describes it. Both parties resort to using vague terms such as *down there*. This avoidance only serves to perpetuate an image of female sexuality as dark and mysterious. Having a limited vocabulary may put women at risk of inadequately describing or asking questions about their genitalia. Furthermore, women's sexual problems may not be adequately addressed due to these evasions.

Education is Key

A combination of different education resources is recommended in improving sexual health literacy, such as:

- Exposing women to photographs showing a wide array of vulvas that have not undergone genital cosmetic surgery.

- Giving women accurate information about the function of the vulva and vagina.

- Informing women as to what female genital cosmetic surgery involves, including the risks associated with such procedures.

- Providing information about all aspects of vulvar anatomy, including the biology and physiology of female sexual arousal.

- Exposing women to educational videos has been found to be a useful tool in increasing women's media literacy and awareness of female genital diversity.

- Providing knowledge about the *unreal* media depictions of female genitals due to digital alteration.

- Increasing body/genital awareness and overall sexual functioning through the intervention of mindfulness-based cognitive therapy combined with psycho-sexual-education.

These strategies have been found to have a positive effect on women's genital image and sexual self-esteem.

Barbie Doll Vulval Ideal

It is *NOT* a Barbie World!

Women of all ages are expressing concerns about the appearance of their vulva to their doctors. This increase of genital image anxiety has been attributed to pubic hair grooming practices to particularly those that remove all pubic hair through Brazilian waxing and permanent LASER hair removal. The Brazilian has migrated from pornography to the preferred aesthetic of many everyday girls and women. These trends have created a social and cultural view of women's genitals – one which resembles a Barbie doll. A Barbie doll does not have a vulva and some girls have grown up thinking their adult vulva will look like Barbie's. Perhaps a Barbie doll with pubic hair would be too confronting for many. Not for me – growing up I didn't have a Barbie doll of my own, but as a grown woman I am the proud owner of *Feral Cheryl,* an anti-Barbie doll.

Women pluck, tweeze, shave, scrape, shock or LASER away pubic hair according to the latest fashion trends which are also attributed to images women see in the media. Pubic hair coiffing ensures women are more involved in an anxious self-scrutiny of their genitals. Women's attention is then drawn to the size and shape of their labia minora and a distortion as to what women perceive as *normal* arises. What was normal before the removal of pubic hair is now considered to be abnormal when the mons pubis and labia majora are exposed.

Having a hairless pubis allows others, such as beauticians who specialise in intimate grooming or a sexual partner, to view and inspect women's genitalia more closely. They may offer recommendations or opinions towards the appearance of women's genitalia, which is sometimes judgemental or disparaging. Such scrutiny by others about something so personal as one's genitals may also lead women to feel greater insecurity with their appearance.

Cosmetic Surgery & the Vulval Ideal

The cosmetic surgery industry has promoted the Barbie doll vulval ideal. For example, some cosmetic surgeons offer women the *opportunity* to have their labia minora trimmed or removed so their vulva can be portrayed as prepubescent, round, smooth with no visible labia minora. The popularity of the total removal of pubic hair has also made the Barbie doll-look desirable. The problem with the Barbie doll vulval ideal is that women who are worried about their genital appearance may be vulnerable to seeking out altering their *normal* genital appearance. Women want to have an ideal vulva that has been created and marketed to them. The popularity of female genital cosmetic surgery has been promoted aggressively by many cosmetic surgery clinics.

Women who choose female genital cosmetic surgery are seemingly brainwashed by societal attitudes about genital normality and hoodwinked by certain surgeons who perform female genital cosmetic surgery that these procedures are relatively quick and risk-free. One extremely powerful strategy that some cosmetic surgeons use is the publication of before and after photographs to promote their image of the vulval ideal what they (mostly male surgeons) deem to be a shift from the imperfect to the *perfect* vulva. These clinics aim to generate business and expose women to images of an *ideal* vulva – that is, one which is not visible. Women make negative comparisons with their own and other women's genitals based on the presented before and after images.

Choice is an Illusion

Another strategy, perhaps the most powerful one in my view, is the rhetoric that many cosmetic surgeons are purportedly only giving women what they want. Women are being deceived under the guise of women's choice. This is the rhetoric used by many surgeons in justifying their business plan. I am the first to agree that women are able to do whatever they choose with their bodies. If you choose to undergo, or have already undergone, some type of genital cosmetic surgery, that is absolutely all right. I respect the rights of adult women to undergo female genital cosmetic surgery subject to informed consent, which includes appropriate education.

What I am espousing here is that some surgeons who perform female genital cosmetic surgery are not fully informing women about the procedures and their side effects. They do not provide women with *all* the information, including other options and opinions, women are unable to make an individualised and informed choice and give valid consent for the cosmetic surgery that they may otherwise *choose* to undergo. Consent must be fully informed for women to be empowered to make a meaningful decision. Women are misinformed by the empty promises of what genital cosmetic surgery will give them, such as vulval beauty and sexual enhancement. The industry hides behind the catchcry of empowering women's lives. Be fooled no more. These marketing strategies do not constitute empowerment for women. Rather, they represent a devious medical deception.

Case in point is the appropriation by some female genital cosmetic surgeons of a medical condition called *hypertrophy*. The condition of *hypertrophy of the labia minora* has not been defined in the field of medicine. Hypertrophy of the labia minora is a pseudo-medical condition dreamed up by the cosmetic industry. It is used to legitimise cosmetic labia minora reduction surgery and has turned a normal variation in vulval appearance into a *real* medical problem, as discussed below.

In 2011 I attended a congress in Las Vegas organised by the International Society of Cosmetogynecology (ISCG) called *World Congress on Female & Male Cosmetic Genital Surgery*. As one of the token female presenters at this conference, it felt like I was walking into the lion's den. It was essentially a public relations event showcasing high profile genital cosmetic surgeons, some of whom had reached celebrity status. Many were eager to put their name to yet another surgical technique. The congress was basically a club where certain surgeons, predominantly men met and discussed marketing strategies on how to make a profit from cutting, amputating, injecting, snipping, burning and sucking away at women's healthy and normal genitalia.

Dr Lindy McDougall, a medical anthropologist, who also attended the Las Vegas conference, has written a profound exposé of the convergence of the medical (surgeons') gaze on women's genitalia and consequent female genital cosmetic surgeries. In *The Perfect Vagina* McDougall delivers insights into the upsurgence of female genital cosmetic surgery and relays the experiences and opinions of both surgeons and their patients.

HYPERTROPHY

PSEUDO-MEDICAL CONDITION OR MEDICAL FRAUD?

In the case of labia minora reduction cosmetic surgery (labiaplasty), hypertrophy is a medical word used by cosmetic surgeons to create a problem for women that does not exist. In their efforts to sell women the perfect vulva and vagina, it has been argued that cosmetic surgery clinics are promoting genital image anxiety among women. Health professionals are concerned about the increased number of women seeking labiaplasty, as there has been no known increase in labial dimensions over the last thirty years. Women's normal and natural genital diversity has been turned into a medical problem. Essentially, cosmetic surgery clinics are touting that the normal bodily variations that exist between women are abnormal. This, of course, is not true. Cosmetic surgery clinics do not care if your vulva is of normal variation – they are in the business of making money and seek to capitalise out of women's genital anxieties.

A common marketing strategy used by some cosmetic surgery clinics is *upselling*. Upselling is presenting for one procedure, for instance, labiaplasty (labia minora reduction) and told that you could benefit from a clitoral hood reduction, along with G-spot augmentation. No need to worry about paying upfront, as the charming consultant can arrange a payment plan or encourage you to access your favourite buy-now and pay-later mobile app. Upselling simply brings more financial profit to the particular cosmetic surgeon. You don't even have to visit a clinic in-person as some websites offer online consultations with the option of uploading an image of your genitals.

Many cosmetic surgeons have arguably cashed in on promoting the *condition* of not having a pretty vulva. Cosmetic surgery clinics capitalise on this so-called condition by portraying inherently risky procedures as an unproblematic way for women to achieve a *perfect* looking and *super* sexual functioning vulva and vagina. In this way, a fateful cycle has been created as clinics pathologise female genital diversity.

Cookie Cutter Aesthetics

Female genital cosmetic surgery becomes a practice of changing women's diverse bodies to fit a certain (male-oriented) aesthetic of what women's genitals should look like ...

– Dr Virginia Braun

I totally support the premise of free sexual expression. However, some women are very uncomfortable with the so-called sexual freedom and choices put to them. Choosing drastic cosmetic surgery can cause more problems as many women are very disappointed with the results.

So, is it men or women who want vulvas to be of a cookie cutter aesthetic? In short, the answer is both. However, the answer is far more complex as there are several sociocultural influences that contribute to the increase in genital image anxiety. Having a vulva that looks like your Barbie doll when you were a child or looking like the women you and your sexual partner see in pornography will almost certainly never guarantee you a happier sex life. Female genital cosmetic surgery is not the antidote to improving an unhealthy relationship.

There is no such thing as *normal* – there is only *diversity*, where every woman's vulva is different. What we do know is that everyone's body size and shape are not the same and that each one of us looks unique. So being different is normal. It is helpful to think that the features of our vulva are all different. No vulva is identical to another women's vulva. The appearance of every woman's vulva is unique – vulvas come in all different shapes, colours and sizes.

The issue is that there are several sociocultural reasons that have contributed to genital image anxieties. Furthermore, the increase in women wanting to have female genital cosmetic surgery indicates that some women may mistakenly believe that sexual satisfaction is dependent on the anatomical appearance of their genitals. They may seek out cosmetic surgery to improve their sexual relationship. However, female genital cosmetic surgery is not a magic cure-all.

Congratulations, *Vulva Image Warrior!* This is the end of this section of your journey of discovering the sociocultural issues that have given rise to genital image troubles and anxieties. The next section will firstly reflect on the evolution of female genital cosmetic surgery. Secondly, the different types of female genital cosmetic surgery and their associated risks will be evaluated. Finally, the motivations of why some women would choose to have female genital cosmetic surgery will be explored.

V-SECTION THREE

The Ugly Truth About Female Genital Cosmetic Surgery

Cosmetic surgery culture promotes the very anxieties it seeks to quell.

– Anthony Elliott

Women's bodies feature publicly as if they are the central focus of our lives, denying our humanity as whole human beings. From our foreheads to our toes, from our collar bones to our fingertips, from the crowns of our heads to the intimacy of our vulva, women's bodies are sites to be shaped by forces outside our control. Divided into body parts, swathed in the plastic of performance, women continue to be denied personhood.

– Jocelynne A. Scutt

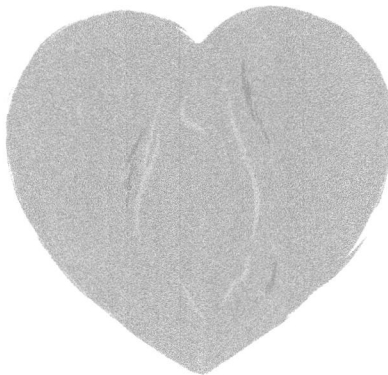

SURGERY ON WOMEN'S GENITALIA IS NOTHING NEW

Female genital cosmetic surgery refers to cosmetic surgical procedures performed on the healthy external genitalia of cisgender women, or internally in the case of G-spot amplification, hymen reconstruction and vaginal tightening. Female genital cosmetic surgery is not genital surgery that is undertaken to treat medical conditions, such as *genitourinary cancer, vulvar cancer, congenital adrenal hyperplasia* or *chronic vulvar irritation*; nor does it refer to *vaginoplasty*, which is a medical surgery to create a vagina during intersex or male-to-female sex-reassignment surgery or to repair major genital anomalies. Additionally, female genital cosmetic surgery does not refer to female genital mutilation/cutting, a highly controversial body modification procedure that is concentrated in Africa, the Middle East and Asia but is prohibited in Australia.

Surgery on women's genitalia is not new. Between the nineteenth and mid-twentieth centuries, surgeons performed *clitoridectomies* (removal or reduction of the clitoris) on women and girls as a therapy to control *deviant* sexual behaviour, such as the solitary act of masturbation, non-heterosexuality and hypersexuality. *Clitoral hood reductions* (*circumcisions*) were also performed on married women so they were able to have orgasms more easily with their husband. These surgeries were used to control and redirect women's sexual behaviour and were considered appropriate medical treatment at the time.

The surgical practice of altering women's genitalia continues today as part of a range of female genital cosmetic surgical techniques. Female genital cosmetic surgery is about normalising the female body, so the appearance and function of women's genitals are in alignment with the norms and standards of the dominant heterosexist culture. The paradoxical heterosexist view of women's sexuality is where men desire women with prepubescent external genitalia or vulvas, who simultaneously have the capacity to be more receptive to orgasm during penetrative sex.

The Evulva-Lution of Female Genital Cosmetic Surgery

The term *designer vagina* first emerged out of medical surgical procedures to repair episiotomies or spontaneous tears after childbirth, which were routinely performed in this context since the 1950s. The surgery involves repairing these tears with stiches. An overzealous repair, using the notorious *husband stitch*, is an extra stitch performed by some doctors to tighten a women's vagina after childbirth and is, in some instances, performed with the stated intention of improving women's sexual health and wellbeing. An extra stitch to tighten the vagina post-birth may result in some women experiencing sexual pleasure. However, the surgery is highly controversial and may result in the woman experiencing sexual pain (*introital dyspareunia*), rather than pleasure. Many researchers argue that the husband stitch is performed to increase the male partner's sexual pleasure, not the female partner's. The routine practice of episiotomy was an accepted medical practice for many years. Today, episiotomies are no longer routinely performed in Australia and are only done with the woman's consent or in a genuine emergency.

Labiaplasty (labia minora reduction) was first described in the scientific literature in 1976. Owing to aggressive advertising and marketing campaigns by surgeons involved in performing cosmetic surgeries on women's genitalia in the late-1990s and early-2000s, the term *designer vagina* emerged in the popular vernacular to describe female genital cosmetic surgery.

The term *vaginal rejuvenation* is another umbrella term for female genital cosmetic surgery which emerged around the late 1990s. The term has caused confusion among patients because surgeons use it inconsistently to describe different types of procedures and there is no agreement on what vaginal rejuvenation actually is. Rejuvenation is defined as *making more youthful*, the aim of many genital cosmetic surgical procedures.

This lack of consistent terminology is pervasive in the genital cosmetic surgery industry. There is no standardisation of nomenclature for labelling different types of surgeries. On the contrary, there is an array of terms associated with the same surgical procedures which have evolved from advertising and marketing strategies and not from evidenced-based practice or medicine.

Female genital cosmetic surgery is also known by myriad names including, but not limited to:

cosmetogynecology, cosmetic genitoplasty, external genitalia rejuvenation, genital beautification, vulvovaginal aesthetic surgery, vaginal rejuvenation, vulvovaginal plastic surgery, cosmetic vulvar surgery, aesthetic genital surgery, genital rejuvenation and female genital plastic surgery.

The cosmetic surgery industry is constantly evolving and developing new female genital cosmetic surgery names and techniques.

The vulva and vagina consist of a cluster of intimately related anatomical structures that are the center of women's sexual function. Many of the female genital cosmetic surgeries are not evidenced based. Researchers today have only just begun to map female genital anatomy and are making new discoveries on how the different structures are connected. This research is groundbreaking in redefining women's sexuality and rewriting the anatomy books.

Female Genital Cosmetic Surgery: The Last Frontier

For decades women have been able to have every aspect of their face altered through cosmetic surgery. The menu of cosmetic surgery alterations to the face includes altering the nose (*rhinoplasty*), eyelids (*blepharoplasty*), chin (*mentoplasty*), ears (*otoplasty*), face (*rhytidectomy/meloplasty*) and injecting dermal fillers to their chin, lips, cheeks and forehead. So too every aspect of the vulval anatomy can be changed through some type of female cosmetic surgery. You may have heard about the cosmetic procedure on the labia minora called *labiaplasty* as this is the most common procedure performed on women's genitalia in Australia. From the surgeons who perform these procedures, female genital cosmetic surgery is the last frontier of the women's body to be altered by their scalpel or LASER.

Many doctors, psychologists, sexual health counsellors and researchers are alarmed and concerned by why women who have normal genitals would seek out female genital cosmetic surgery to alter their genital appearance. One of the main issues concerning female genital cosmetic surgery is that it is being performed on women who have normal genitals. Another concern is that female genital cosmetic surgery can impair women's sexual functioning. Components of the vulva have two types of vascular tissue – *erectile* and *non-erectile*. Each having their own specialised as well as their unified response to sexual arousal. Any disruption made on these structures through cosmetic surgery can potentially have detrimental effects on women's sexuality.

DIMENSIONS OF GENITAL IMAGE AND WOMEN'S DESIRE TO UNDERGO FEMALE GENITAL COSMETIC SURGERY

Female genital image research is a relatively new area of female body image research. Broadly speaking, there are three dimensions of genital image:

Genital satisfaction is an evaluation of the appearance of one's genitals. This dimension of genital image captures how much women are satisfied or dissatisfied with the overall appearance of their vulva as well as the appearance of specific aspects of their vulva. For instance, how satisfied or dissatisfied one is with the size of their labia minora or the overall attractiveness of their vulva.

Genital self-image is an evaluation of emotional reactions to one's genital appearance and function. This dimension of genital image refers to women's feelings and emotions about their genitals. For instance, how anxious, confident, shameful, self-conscious or embarrassed one feels about their genitals.

Genital image in the bedroom is a dimension of genital image that captures how self-conscious women are about their body and genitals during sexual activity. For instance, how self-conscious one partner feels about the other partner looking at their genitals during sexual activity.

Researchers have found that women who have negative genital image (dissatisfied with their appearance of their genitals and/or have poor genital self-image and/or are self-conscious about their body/genitals in the sexual setting) were more interested in undergoing some type of female genital cosmetic surgery than women with a positive genital image. Health professionals are increasingly concerned about the rising numbers of women seeking some form of female genital cosmetic surgery.

The following pages will shed light on the low standard of evidence for and the risks associated with female genital cosmetic surgery.

Types of Female Genital Cosmetic Surgery

The different parts of the female genital anatomy that can be altered by *cosmetic* surgery include the labia minora, labia majora, mons pubis, introitus (vaginal opening), clitoral hood, walls of the vagina and hymen. Broadly speaking, there are nine categories of procedures: *labia minora reduction, labia majora augmentation, mons pubis and labia majora reduction, vaginal tightening, clitoral hood reduction, clitoral repositioning, G-spot amplification, hymen reconstruction* and *energy-based vaginal procedures.*

It is very important to understand not only about how your genitals function but what might happen if you decide to alter some part of your vulval anatomy through female genital cosmetic surgery. We will be looking at the motivations for women choosing female genital cosmetic surgery. We will also be exploring the potential psychological and physical risks associated with having female genital *cosmetic* surgery.

How Many Australian Women Are Having Female Genital Cosmetic Surgery?

It is currently unclear how many female genital cosmetic procedures are currently being performed in Australia. The main reason for this is that female genital cosmetic surgery is elective and is not covered by Australia's publicly funded healthcare system – the Medicare Benefits Scheme. Since 2014, women can only claim through Medicare if the surgery performed on the vulva is deemed to be medically indicated. That is that the women have a structural abnormality that is causing her significant functional impairment. It is also deemed to be medically indicated for women to be able to claim through Medicare if the women's labium extends more than 8cm below the vaginal introitus while she is in a standing position.

Before 2014, Medicare data indicated that the number of female genital cosmetic surgery procedures were trending upwards. Since the 2014 changes by Medicare there has been a marked decline in the number of procedures funded with approximately 81 procedures carried out annually for medically indicated reasons. Before the 2014 changes a total of 9,864 procedures were performed with an average of 1,409 procedures performed per year (2007-2014). The figures prior to the 2014 changes indicate that female genital procedures were largely for cosmetic or aesthetic reasons and were not performed for a clear medical need under Medicare. We have to turn to the international data to see how the figures are trending. These indicate that year after year, the number of women having labiaplasties has been increasing, not only in Australia but globally.

Most cosmetic surgeries, including female genital cosmetic surgery, are carried out by surgeons in the private health sector in Australia where the industry is largely unregulated and unaudited. In this context, female genital cosmetic surgery is performed by a range of practitioners, including plastic surgeons, cosmetic doctors and gynaecologists. Currently, it is legal for doctors with a basic medical degree and no formal specialist surgical training to perform cosmetic surgery in Australia. This lack of regulation potentially puts women seeking genital cosmetic surgery at risk from practitioners who are not professionally trained.

Equally troubling is the lack of evidence-based data concerning the outcomes of female genital cosmetic surgery in Australia. This raises a public health risk as no scientific research or statistics are available to evaluate the safety and efficacy of different types of procedures and associated techniques and the long-term impact and implications that these may have on women's health and wellbeing. Labiaplasty has been reported to be the world's fastest growing cosmetic surgery procedure. Accordingly, the reasons why women seek this procedure are more extensively reported in the literature than for any other type of female genital cosmetic surgery.

Women of all ages are expressing concerns about the appearance of their vulva. Some women have reported that they have not been sexually active and are wanting cosmetic surgery to help with their sexual self-esteem. Being dissatisfied with one's genital appearance is not something that is appropriately addressed through female genital cosmetic surgery. Australian health professionals are especially concerned as they are seeing rising rates of young women in their twenties, teens and even as young as their tweens with genital image anxiety and wanting to alter their genitalia. The younger the woman is at the time of her first labiaplasty, the more likely it is that she will need further labiaplasties to maintain the desired ideal aesthetic in future.

Risks & Reasons

Does Female Genital Cosmetic Surgery Upgrade or Downgrade Women's Bodies & Sexuality?

We have covered the varied sociocultural reasons behind why women would undergo unnecessary genital cosmetic surgery on their normal and healthy genitalia. Now, let's explore in more detail what is involved in the different types of surgeries and the potential risks, as well as the functional (physical) and non-functional (psychological) motivations for women choosing female genital cosmetic surgery.

Cosmetic Surgery on the Labia Minora

Labiaplasty is a procedure that makes the labia minora smaller, reducing the size (length and/or width) of the labia minora (either bilaterally or unilaterally). By removing part of the labia minora this can also make the clitoral glans more prominent.

It is difficult to identify distinct techniques used in the procedure, as surgeons often do not provide detailed descriptions of what the various surgeries entail. Procedures broadly fall into two categories:

- **Amputation** – involves trimming the free edge of the labia minora. A strip of the labia minora are excised or amputated to the desired size and then oversewn. This technique is known to cause scarring of the newly revised free edge.

- **Section removal** – involves the removal of a section of the labia minora. This is a more complex procedure than the simple amputation and includes cutting away a V-shaped or W-shaped section of the labium minora, then suturing the labium together again.

These procedures have not been evaluated comparatively. The wedge resection technique is said to be superior cosmetically, but it carries higher risk of complications.

Labiaplasty is known by numerous names, including:

labioplasty, labia minora reduction, minoroplasty, labial hypertrophy, labia design, vaginal labiaplasty, vaginal lip reduction, labial rejuvenation, reconstruction labioplasty, nymphectomy, nymphoplasty, labial reduction, combination labiaplasty, expert labiaplasty, fenestration labiaplasty, fenestration labioreduction, labioreduction, LASER reduction labiaplasty, LASER reduction labioplasty, designer LASER labiaplasty, pubisplasty, stem-iris labial sculpting, labial reduction beautification, labial correction, labial vontouring and *LASER vaginal rejuvenation®*, which is trademarked by United States gynaecologist, Dr Matlock.

There are myriad names for labiaplasty techniques. It appears that each surgeon wants to make their mark on the industry to attain a marketing edge. Could it be *ego-based practice* more than *medical evidence-based practice*? Perhaps to get ahead in the industry, cosmetic surgeons are dreaming-up new names and techniques to impress and lure women. '*Will it be a rim or a Barbie?*' is the catchcry of one leading cosmetic surgeon. The signature labiaplasty he refers to as a *rim* procedure is where just the edge of the inner labia is left, whereas the signature *Barbie* procedure is where the entire inner labia minora is cut off!

There are many labiaplasty techniques referred to as:

> *Simple labioplasty (involves partial or full amputation of entire labium with oversewing), W-shaped resection, running W-shape resection, lazy S-shaped resection, central V-wedge, central wedge with hockey-stick resection, zig-zag labiaplasty, W-plasty, star labiaplasty (modified double wedge resection), inferior V-plasty reduction, central wedge nymphectomy with a 90 degree Z-plasty, inferior wedge resection, superior pedicle flap reconstruction, Ostrzenski's fenestration labiaplasty with inferior flap transposition, de-epithelialised reductive labiaplasty techniques, LASER labiaplasty, lambda LASER nymphoplasty, extended wedge resection labiaplasty, edge trim labiaplasty, free-edge or edge resection labiaplasty, horseshoe labiaplasty, custom flask labiaplasty, curved linear resection, posterior wedge resection techniques, composite reduction labiaplasty, the rim, the barbie, the hybrid and the peek-a-boo.*

Who knew that such a small part of the female genital anatomy could attract so much attention! This *word salad* of procedures just causes confusion among women who are trying to navigate this messy area of pseudo-medical practice.

Understanding Why Women Seek Labiaplasty

The reasons why women seek to undergo labiaplasty (or any type of female genital cosmetic surgery) are complex and varied and heavily influenced by a range of sociocultural factors. Understanding the *why* will assist us in supporting women who are considering undergoing a potentially risky and unnecessary procedure on their normal and healthy genitalia.

1. **The labia minora protrude beyond the edge of their labia majora –** The most common non-functional complaint of women who seek labiaplasty is dissatisfaction with the appearance of their labia minora. Some women experience sexual or social embarrassment if their labia minora protrude beyond the edge of their labia majora. You may notice that on some of the surgeons' websites they refer to this protrusion as *hypertrophy*. Some health experts and researchers note that the medical and scientific literature do not agree on what constitute normal dimensions of the labia minora. Protruding labia

minora are a normal bodily variation for women. It is not a malformation or even unusual. For some women they are unaware of this normal variation and consider their labia minora abnormal.

2. **The labia minora are lacking symmetry** – Another common non-functional complaint is from women who are concerned their labia minora are not symmetrical. Some women want their labia minora to be the same size and shape to fit the ideal genital image. A further complaint concerns colouration of the edges of the labia minora, which tend to darken around the time of adolescence or during pregnancy. Adolescence and pregnancy are reproductive milestones and hyperpigmentation to the labia minora occurs naturally at that time due to increases in hormonal levels. Some women are dissatisfied with the darker colour of the skin on the edges of their labia minora and want it to be paler to appear more youthful. In reality, there is great variation between women's labia minora shape, symmetry and skin colouration.

3. **Psychological reasons** – Often women who seek labiaplasty or some type of female genital cosmetic surgery want to address their low self-esteem, body shame, anxiety, depression, embarrassment, mood disturbances and other psychological symptoms.
   - **Self-consciousness** – Some women feel self-conscious about their body and/or their genital appearance during sexual activity and avoid sexual practices such as oral sex, masturbation and intercourse.
   - **Sexual trauma** – If a woman has experienced childhood sexual abuse and/or sexual assault this may damage their body image resulting in bodily shame about the appearance of

women's genitals. Some women may seek out labiaplasty to reclaim this part of their body.

4. **Domestic violence –** This is a social issue and is very common for women to experience. Women may be harassed or coerced by their intimate partner to undergo labiaplasty or some other type of female genital cosmetic surgery. Some women are *urged* by their male sexual partner/s to have labiaplasty to satisfy their male partner's sexual proclivities.

5. **Relationship issues –** Some women have the expectation that labiaplasty will improve their sex life, whilst other women may believe it will save their marriage or relationship.

6. **Teased or bullied –** Women who are dissatisfied with the appearance of their labia minora may have had a negative experience or received negative commentary about their genitals by their current partner, former sexual partner/s, friend or peers, a family member, a medical professional or a sexual abuse or sexual assault perpetrator. Some women are dissatisfied with the appearance of their labia minora after hearing negative commentary or disparaging jokes about other women's genitals.

7. **Purely aesthetic reasons –** The motivation for some women to have labiaplasty is purely aesthetic. They are dissatisfied with the appearance of their labia minora. Some women:
   - feel restricted in their clothing choices and are self-conscious that their labia minora are visible when they wear tight fitting clothing
   - express concern about starting a new sexual relationship due to their anxiety about the appearance of their labia minora

It has been reported by the medical profession that young women and girls have been presenting with concerns about the appearance of their genitals and are in some instances requesting to have their labia minora reduced. A considerable number of these young women and girls present to medical clinics and children's hospitals with anxiety about the appearance of their labia minora. Some young women are brought in by their mothers who are concerned about the appearance of their daughter's genitalia.

Performing labiaplasty on a young, developing body could risk nerve damage, scarring, narrowing of the introitus (vaginal opening) and interfere with future sexual arousal and satisfaction. Female genital cosmetic surgery for non-medical reasons on female children and adolescents, whose external genitals are not fully developed, is not only unethical but illegal under current legislation in all Australian states including the Crimes (Female Genital Mutilation) Act 1996 of Victoria (Crimes [Female Genital Mutilation] Act 1996.

8. **Maternal concerns** – Some mothers are worried about the appearance of their tween and teen daughters' labia minora. Some mothers may not understand the changes that occur during puberty for their daughters. Children's bodies are in a constant state of growth and some significant changes occur during their tween and teen years. Puberty and the development of the vulva can start at different times throughout these years:
    *   It is very common for a girl's labia minora to develop before the labia majora develops.
    *   The labia minora develop during the tween years between the ages of 8 and 12.
    *   On a thin girl the labia minora can appear to be more prominent.
    *   The labia majora develop during the teenage years between the ages of 13 and 19.

- Everyone is different down there – and different is normal.

Some mothers have told me they became concerned when teaching their daughters how to use tampons. For many teens it is quite the norm to remove all their pubic hair – which just makes everything else more visible to the naked eye. Some mothers consult Dr Google which immediately directs their search to cosmetic surgery websites. The misinformation on the websites heightens mother's fears.

This is all well-meaning, and many women have a limited knowledge of genital image diversity. The database we have of how a labia minora should look like is very limited. After all, not many women have seen their own vulva let alone the vulva of other females. Tweens' and teens' vulvas do not look the same as their mother's. Fortunately, many mothers seek the advice of doctors. Once it is explained to them that these vulval changes are a normal and natural part of the developmental process, many mums and their daughters are reassured. Others, however, will go ahead and have the surgery regardless of any reassurance.

I am often asked by mothers how they can emotionally support their tween and teen daughters in navigating their way through this developmental stage of their life. Mothers can help to promote self-acceptance and reassurance in their tween or teen daughters by explaining that the changes that are happening to their body are normal. Here is a booklet with important stuff about *Girls and Puberty* you could share with your teenager. Mothers can also support them through educational genital image diversity awareness and emphasising that their body and their vulva is normal. Mothers who have daughters who want to undergo labiaplasty need to explain to their daughters that surgery may not help her to achieve a standard of ideal vulval beauty. Surgery may remove vulval sensation and sensitivity. Surgery is not psychotherapy and will not address the underlying emotional concerns that give rise to distress over genital appearance.

Labiaplasties are being performed in increasing rates among girls and adolescents in Australia, as well as in other countries. Similarly on the rise are the numbers of mothers who are talking to doctors and gynaecologists about their concerns in relation to the appearance and changes they have observed in their daughter's labia minora. These increases indicate that mothers are not being given the correct information about the changes that occur to the vulva during puberty and are therefore not able to pass this knowledge onto their daughters. Perhaps some mothers did not have sufficient sexual education about normal genital appearance when they were growing up. If you are a mother with concerns, please go and have a talk with your GP on your own before including your daughter. Many mums have been reassured by their doctor after having a conversation about their concerns regarding the developmental changes expected for girls.

A young girl's body is still undergoing pubertal development and growth – the changes to her labia minora may not be completed until early adulthood. If the psychosocial issues and genital diversity awareness education have not been explored with young girls, it may certainly catapult her into further unhappiness. If genital image concerns are not appropriately addressed, the surgery may make young girls feel worse and not better. The cosmetic, or aesthetic, result of having undergone alteration of the labia minora through labiaplasty is not permanent. This is due to the genital anatomy changes women will experience over their lifespan such as pregnancy and menopause. Each time a woman has the surgery there are increased risks of scarring and loss of sensitivity to her labia minora.

9. **Body dysmorphic disorder –** Some women who seek labiaplasty for non-functional reasons experience body dysmorphic disorder. Body dysmorphic disorder is a type of obsessive-compulsive disorder. Someone with body dysmorphia is excessively preoccupied with a perceived or slight defect in their appearance which causes them significant distress or impairment in their daily functioning. The prevalence of body dysmorphic disorder is more common in cosmetic surgery populations than in the general population.

10. **Sexual pleasure –** One common functional reason for some women seeking labiaplasty is to enhance their sexual responsiveness and/or to enhance the sexual responsiveness of their male partner. This echoes the reason why some surgeons perform the controversial husband stitch, which is purported to enhance the sexual pleasure of women's male sexual partners.

11. **Pain or discomfort –** There are also functional complaints that prompt some women to seek labiaplasty for ostensibly medical reasons. Concerns identified by surgeons focus largely on pain or discomfort relating to the size of the labia minora. For instance, some women experience:
    - difficulty in vaginal penetration or entry dyspareunia (sexual pain) due to invagination of protuberant labia minora tissue during sexual activity
    - difficulty with indwelling urethral catheters
    - difficulty maintaining vaginal hygiene
    - chronic irritation
    - pain or discomfort with wearing tight clothing
    - pain or discomfort with exercise when riding a bicycle or a horse

Medicare now distinguishes between cosmetic and medically indicated reasons for undergoing labiaplasty. Women who have a medical need to reduce the size of their labia minora are required to undergo a functional assessment to access the public health system.

12. **Functional and non-functional reasons** – Finally, some women present with both functional and non-functional complaints. For instance, a woman may feel self-conscious about the appearance of her labia minora and this, in turn, interferes with her comfort during sex. The woman is not able to become sufficiently aroused and consequently experiences dyspareunia (sexual pain). She seeks labiaplasty in an effort to improve her sex life and sexual self-esteem. Interestingly, some women report a lack of sexual desire after having undergone labiaplasty.

As you can see, there are many reasons why women have labiaplasty. *Centrefold* is an award-winning animated documentary exploring the personal accounts of three women who have had labiaplasty.

Your Labia Minora

A Highly Sensitive Sexual Organ

The labia minora are highly innervated which means they are highly sensitive. This fragile sexual organ also contains erectile tissue, which plays an important role in women's sexual response. Having a labiaplasty means that valuable sensory and erotic tissue is removed. There is no way to put it back – once it is gone, it is gone! Removing the labia minora can alter or reduce sexual function. Some women who have had labiaplasty report experiencing reduced sensitivity and sexual pleasure during sexual activity. The labia minora are in very close proximity to the clitoral hood. During sexual arousal the labia minora increase in size and this engorgement stimulates the clitoris. Labiaplasty risks this interconnectedness between the labia minora and clitoris. Any alteration potentially reduces the potency of this important sexual organ.

Your Labia Minora and Vulvovaginal Health

The labia minora also play an important role in maintaining vulvovaginal health. As mentioned earlier, the labia minora enclose and protect the urethral opening and inner parts of the vagina from infection. The labia minora also assist in directing the urine stream while voiding. Health professionals warn that having the labia minora removed could change the sexual function and the health and hygiene of the vulva.

Botched: Risks and Complications

It is difficult to find surgeons who readily report the number of labiaplasty complications that women experience at their hands. However, it has been reported that adolescents who have labiaplasty experience more post-op complications than adult women. Women of all ages who undergo labiaplasty may experience several complications such as vaginal dryness, scar tenderness, discomfort from wearing underwear and urinary voiding problems. Some adolescents have noticed since the operation that the size of their labia minora has grown. This growth may be due to hormonal changes to the labia minora and vulva that occur during adolescent development. Anecdotal reports suggest that some women who have a vaginal delivery when giving birth after labiaplasty may be at higher risk of an episiotomy or labial and vaginal tears than women who have not undergone this procedure. Rigorous evidence-based research concerning the outcomes of labiaplasty and vaginal delivery is needed.

Aside from causing serious functional problems, labiaplasty may also result in permanent disfigurement, including a hole in the labia, necrosis, scar tissue formation, haematoma (clot formation), infections, dyspareunia, hypersensitivity, chronic vulvar pain, repair separation, bleeding and wound management issues. Other functional problems include loss of sensation that can result in difficulty in arousal and anorgasmia. Disfigurement and pain can cause great distress, resulting in an aversion to sexual activity, depression and suicidal ideation has been reported in some women. As more labiaplasties are performed, women who are dissatisfied with the appearance of their labia minora post-surgery may seek revision surgery to rectify the resulting disfigurement or aesthetic problem.

Little, if any, information is provided by cosmetic surgeons on their websites regarding the short-term and long-term risks of surgery. The marketing is prolific with numerous unsubstantiated claims and erroneous information of the enduring physical, psychological and sexual benefits to the unsuspecting public.

The studies that have examined patient satisfaction and psychological outcomes of women who have had labiaplasty are inconclusive. Some women may be satisfied with the appearance and function of their labia minora post-surgery while others may experience greater physical or psychological distress. For the latter group, labiaplasty may create problems that were non-existent prior to the procedure.

Cosmetic labiaplasty procedures raise ethical issues and post-surgery risks that are all too serious for professional bodies to continue to ignore. While some women self-reported they benefited initially, it is unknown if the physical, psychological and sexual functioning effects, both positive and negative, are enduring. Current practices are exceedingly diverse and poorly described in the literature.

Cosmetic Surgery on the Labia Majora

Labia majora augmentation is a cosmetic surgical procedure involving the enlargement of the labia majora. A number of techniques are used to increase the volume of the labia majora include: the *injection of hyaluronic acid filler, lipofilling, dermal fat grafts, autologous fat transfer* and *de-epithelialisation*. Fat transfer techniques include autologous fat grafting, fat injections and lipofilling, which refers to a procedure that uses your own fat that is collected from another area of your body and deposited into the labia majora.

Reasons

There is scant literature on the reasons and motivations for why women seek surgery to increase the size of their labia majora. Some women have, however, reported that they have sought labia majora augmentation as they wanted the area to appear fuller and symmetrical to make it more aesthetically appealing. The surgery can be done for aesthetics as an anti-ageing procedure. The majority of women who have undergone the procedure are in their fifties and have cited their motivation as being the desire to appear more youthful.

The surgery can also be done for functional indications. After having the procedure women have reported having greater comfort during intercourse and increased sexual satisfaction. Surgeons advertise the surgery to women whose labia majora have deflated or lost volume through weight loss, low body fat and ageing (i.e., during menopause, with the decrease in oestrogen, the labia majora often become less prominent) The procedure may also be performed to make the labia majora the desired proportion with the size and shape of the labia minora.

Risks

Labia majora augmentation is experimental and the results of lipofilling and hydraulic acid injections are temporary. Skin grafts, after some time, may be replaced by fibrous tissue. The scientific literature on therapeutic benefits and surgical outcomes is severely lacking. Health professionals are concerned about potential complications from the surgery, as the labia majora play an important role in protecting inner parts of the vulva. The labia majora are sensitive and respond with engorgement during sexual stimulation and arousal and surgical alteration may lead to sexual and functional impairment. Post-operative complications may also include a poor aesthetic result, soft tissue infection, *granuloma*, *haematoma* and *oedema*. Adverse events may also include *flap necrosis* and *pulmonary embolism*.

Cosmetic Surgery on the Mons Pubis and/or Labia Majora

Reduction of the mons pubis and/or labia majora involves the excising of loose skin or the removal of unwanted fat on the mons pubis and/or labia majora through *liposuction*. This surgery is also referred to as *vulvar lipoplasty*. Reduction of the mons pubis is also referred to as *monsplasty, mons lift, pubic lift* or *FUPA lift* (FUPA is an acronym for *Fat Upper Pubic Area*).

Reasons

As with labia majora augmentation surgery, the literature is similarly scant regarding the reasons for why women seek surgery to *reduce* the size of their mons pubis and/or labia majora. The goal of the surgery is purely aesthetic, to flatten the mons pubis and/or labia majora so that women can wear high crotch-fitting and genital hugging clothing. The desired aesthetic also calls for women to denude the area of any sign of pubic hair. Surgeons advertise the surgery to women whose mons pubis and/or labia majora have become prominent due to weight gain, childbirth or as a result of the natural ageing process.

Risks

At the time of writing, no scientific studies exist regarding the safety and effectiveness of reduction of the mons pubis and/or labia majora for cosmetic purposes. The procedure can cause cosmetic irregularities such as skin sagging which may require further cosmetic surgical intervention. The surgical tightening and lifting of underlying muscle and tissue may be required to achieve the desired aesthetic. Post-operative complications may include dyspareunia through over-suction of sub-dermal fat, causing compression pain during sexual activity, as well as infection, bleeding and tenderness.

PERCEPTIONS
OF THE LABIA MAJORA

Why have genital troubles extended to the labia majora? Women may be concerned about changes they have experienced developmentally. For instance, at puberty the mons pubis becomes covered in pubic hair and enlarges due to increased oestrogen. The labia majora are also sensitive to oestrogen at puberty and become enlarged. Women may also become more aware of this area of their genitalia as it is more visible especially when wearing tight clothing. A bulky mons pubis is considered unsightly and has been referred to as a *FUPA*. FUPA is also a slang term that refers to the mons pubis as the *fat upper pussy area*.

Celebrities and models show off their mons pubis and labia majora, sometimes referred to as their *side vagina* while wearing high-cut clothing or sheer material that exposes this area. The labia majora and mons pubis have become highly visible in the media. The ideal vulva is portrayed in the fashion and celebrity media as flat, with no sign of any pubic hair. If one does not have the ideal appearance, this is made a public shame and referred to as having a *camel toe*. *Camel toe* is a slang term that refers to seeing a woman's pudendal cleft through their clothing that accentuates the outer lips (labia majora). This appearance resembles the two toes of a camel's hoof. The labia majora may appear bulky when women wear tight clothes that draw attention to the shape of the outer genitalia which is considered another serious fashion faux pas.

Any nonconformity by women from the ideal vulva is one that delights the media who show these images to publicly shame and humiliate women about their natural, normal bodies. I recently did an internet search and found 51,000,000 results for *camel toe celebrities* that capture headlines such as '*The most shocking cases of celebrity camel toe*' and '*22 worst cases of celebrity camel toe*'. There is social pressure to have a more *pleasing* vulval appearance and a non-surgical solution has been developed. Women can purchase a genital cup/pantiliner protector to wear under their vulva-hugging clothing to hide the ridges of the labia majora and the front lines formed by the pudendal cleft. A technical breakthrough or totally ridiculous? I will let you be the judge.

Camel toe and FUPA are offensive slang terms used to describe the visual effect when women wear a tight-fitting garment around her crotch. The labia majora and mons pubis are both important functional parts of women's genital anatomy and exist as part of women's normal sexual development. Such derogatory comments regarding women's genital appearance and demeaning labelling may be contributing factors as to why women are dissatisfied with the appearance of their labia majora. It seems that women may be negatively influenced via social media and online celebrity news which leads them to feel dissatisfied with their normal vulva, and so they are destined to desire one that conforms to the ideal vulval image.

Cosmetic Surgery on the Vaginal Opening

Vaginal tightening involves the surgical narrowing of the lower third of the vagina. The surgery involves excising portions of the vaginal mucosa using a scalpel, scissors, needle electrode or burning the vaginal wall using a LASER. Other methods involve injecting autologous fat or bulking agents into the vagina.

Reasons

The goal of the surgery is to enhance sexual pleasure for the women and her male sexual partner/s by tightening the women's vagina in order to increase coital friction. Some surgeons market the surgery to women as a type of insurance to prevent their husbands or male partners from being unfaithful. The surgery is associated with virginity and youthfulness and assumes the diameter of a woman's vagina is linked to sexual pleasure.

Risks

The literature on vaginal tightening is limited and no studies have evaluated the safety and effectiveness of the surgery. Due to the lack of evidence-based research and the plethora of techniques adopted by surgeons involved in performing the surgery, the long-term effects are as yet unknown. There is an assumption that the surgery is performed on women who do not have sexual dysfunction. However, there is no data on whether the surgery solves a problem, makes the problem worse or creates a new problem. One such problem is that women who have the surgery before having children may experience obstetric complications when they later become pregnant. There is also a possibility that the surgery may have a positive effect on *vaginal atrophy* (i.e., thinning, drying and inflammation of the vaginal walls due to less oestrogen), but vaginal tightening is experimental in this context and the effects of the surgery are only temporary. It has been documented that, in a rare case, a 34-year-old woman undergoing vaginal tightening died of *non-thrombotic pulmonary embolism* after her vaginal wall was injected with *polyacrylamide hydrogel (PAAG)*. PAAG is a type of filler commonly used for facial contouring and soft tissue augmentation. Non-thrombotic pulmonary embolism is considered to be a serious potential risk of its use.

Cosmetic Surgery on the Vagina using Vaginal LASER Therapy

Vaginal LASER therapy, also called energy-based interventions, is a non-surgical vaginal procedure used to perform *vaginal rejuvenation* (a commercial rather than a scientifically defined term) or vaginal cosmetic procedures to destroy, reshape or tighten the vaginal tissue to change the contour and increase sexual sensation.

There are three types of energy-based devices that are designed to deliver thermal energy to the vaginal wall:

- **Carbon dioxide LASER (CO_2):** The first LASER system to be developed.

- **Erbium-doped yttrium aluminium garnet LASER (Er:YAG):** The second LASER system to be developed.

- **Radiofrequency (RF):** The RF devices work more like microwaves than LASERs and are the most recent system to appear in the *vaginal rejuvenation* market.

The United States Food and Drug Administration (FDA) issued a Safety Communication in 2018 warning women against the use of energy-based devices for treatment of vaginal atrophy and vaginal rejuvenation. The FDA stated these devices have serious risks with concerns around the harm they cause to vaginal skin tissue. Studies have found that LASERs can rejuvenate the hands, face, neck and décolletage areas. However, these devices have insufficient evidence to support their effectiveness in shape-shifting the delicate tissue of the vaginal walls to treat menopausal symptoms, incontinence, reduce sexual pain and vaginal atrophy and laxity. The FDA issued warnings to several companies to cease marketing their devices for vaginal rejuvenation or vaginal cosmetic procedures. Energy-based devices are in the early stages of validation and safety monitoring and therefore there is a need for well-designed studies about the short-term and long-term effects.

Reasons

Cosmetic surgery clinics market energy-based devices to women as non-invasive vaginal tightening and vaginal rejuvenation treatment. They also state this procedure will treat the effects of vaginal atrophy and laxity, correct urinary incontinence, reduce pain during sexual intercourse, treat menopause symptoms and improve sexual function. The devices use similar technology to that of facial rejuvenation which has been modified for vaginal use.

Energy-based interventions are controversial. The FDA warns against using these devices as the health claims are considered deceptive. The FDA wrote letters to several companies about the way these devices have been marketed to vulnerable women, including cancer survivors, without clinical evidence about their safety and effectiveness. These systems are not approved for treating vaginal conditions and yet these and other energy-based devices are available in Australia. There seems to be a never-ending parade of devices are being invented, manufactured and marketed to women as a therapeutic miracle. These devices are being used on women's vaginas without rigorous evidence or standards and are the LASER equivalent of *snake oil*.

Despite these warnings, these devices are extensively marketed in Australia and consumers may not be aware of the controversy around this treatment. These devices are very expensive and may cost the cosmetic surgery clinic $300,000 or more to purchase the lease. When seeking treatment, it is essential for the consumer to be aware of these important health and safety issues. It is very unlikely that clinics will mention these public safety concerns on their websites as the industry is unregulated. Off-label marketing is a widespread issue in the medical field and many of these devices have been marketed for unapproved uses. Further to this, energy-based devices have been used off-label to alter the appearance of the labia minora and labia majora.

LASER DANGER – NOT A MAGIC WAND

Energy-based devices including CO_2 and Erbium LASERs and radiofrequency ablation may cause burns, scarring, pain during sexual intercourse and recurring or chronic vaginal pain. Common adverse events include: *bleeding, spotting, discharge, vulvovaginal pain and/or discomfort, oedema (swelling), dysuria (panful or difficult urination), urinary tract infection, candidiasis, vulvovaginal itching, adhesion formation* and worsening of *dyspareunia.*

Non-Invasive = Pigs Can Fly!

Some women discontinue treatment using energy-based devices due to the discomfort of having the probe inserted into their vagina. It is much like the size of the probe used when having a transvaginal ultrasound. A local anaesthetic cream may be offered and is applied to the vulva. One website states the anaesthetic cream is applied to the probe. The woman's legs are placed in stirrups while the probe is inserted into their vagina, delivering thermal energy into the vaginal tissue and heating the vaginal wall. It is claimed that this treatment plumps up the vaginal wall. Whilst marketed as non-invasive, however, wouldn't this be considered invasive?

Treatment recommendations vary between clinics. One clinic recommended women have three sessions over a period of two months with a further annual maintenance session. Another clinic recommended women have up to five monthly treatments with a further annual maintenance session. The duration of treatment sessions also varies, lasting between 10–20 minutes. The treatment is expensive and costs up to $1,000 per session. This cost to some unsuspecting women is a major concern. The treatment offered by these energy-based devices has not been proven to actually deliver its purported *correction or restoration*. United States urologists, Dr Alexandra Siegal and Dr Barbara M. Chubak (2021) also echo concerns regarding energy-based devices in the management of sexual problems in women as it enters a new era: '*The enthusiasm with which energy-based treatments for sexual dysfunction have been adopted for sale in the medical marketplace is disproportionate to the amount of data that are currently available to support their clinical use.*'

Toothless Tigers & Rogue Elephants

The Australian Therapeutic Goods Administration (TGA) has approved the Erbium:YAG LASER for both tattoo removal and for the treatment of vaginal atrophy. It is unclear as to why this is the case. It is suggested-the Erbium LASER is not as invasive and causes less thermal damage as the other energy-based devices. However, there is not currently any scientific evidence supporting its safety and efficacy and the treatments are not supported for reimbursement under Medicare. Don't you think that when something is described as causing *less* damage that strongly suggests that it is still unsafe? Further, it is important to note that those who operate the devices do not have to have a medical degree.

In Australia, however, these devices are widely available and offered to the unsuspecting public with what appears to be reckless abandon. Perhaps the heavy marketing campaigns that rely on a bombardment of unsubstantiated claims are an effort to recover the enormous costs of purchasing/leasing the equipment. It appears that energy-based devices have slipped through the TGA's regulatory system. Doctors and health professionals want to avoid another trans-vaginal mesh implant scandal that destroyed the health and wellbeing of many Australian women. However, it may be too late. These concerns are echoed throughout the medical profession – you can listen to *MJA* podcast by Dr Melissa Buttini, Consultant Gynaecologist and Professor Christopher Maher, Urogynaecologist, who discuss the potential dangers of energy-based treatment on women's health. These Queensland doctors also make recommendations for safer options to treat symptoms of vulvovaginal atrophy (VVA) and genitourinary syndrome of menopause (GSM). They warn that in light of the FDA response there may be the potential for adverse medico-legal implications for those who continue to use these devices in Australia. Practitioners have a legal obligation to provide patients informed consent and provide sufficient information about risks and side effects of their use and to offer alternative treatment.

THE ANTIDOTE

It is hard to know what the best treatment for menopausal symptoms is on your own. Please consult your health professional regarding the safest and evidenced-based treatment for you. The Jean Hailes Foundation is an Australian not-for-profit organisation that analyses the latest evidence regarding women's health. This resource is well worth having bookmarked on your internet browser.

Confusing Terms & Lack of Scientific Rigour

Some cosmetic surgery websites claim the *rejuvenation* treatment using energy-based devices also tightens the skin (labia) around the vaginal area. It is unclear what part of the female genital anatomy they are referring to. I assume in these instances they are referring to the vaginal opening or introitus – however, this is unclear. It is possible they are referring to the labia minora. They may be *dumbing down* descriptions as they assume women do not know the correct names of their genital anatomy. Not using correct genital anatomy terminology just creates confusion. Unfortunately, using vague and incorrect terminology to describe the site of the women's genital anatomy being altered – aka *rejuvenated* – are not uncommon. Cosmetic surgery websites that list labia tightening as an extra bonus when you undergo vaginal tightening are misleading. These claims are dubious as they have relied on patient testimonials rather than scientific evidence.

WHAT ARE GSM AND VVA?

As you are perusing the websites seeking information about energy-based devices, menopause and women's sexual health, you may come across terms such as *genitourinary syndrome of menopause (GSM)* and *vulvovovaginal atrophy (VVA)*. In 2013 at a consensus conference of the North American Menopause Society and International Society for the Study of Women's Sexual Health (ISSWSH) it was decided a name change was in order. These groups agreed to use the term GSM to more accurately describe the condition previously known as VVA. The choice of the term GSM was to improve communication and management of urogenital and sexual symptoms in post-menopausal women.

GSM refers to:

> ... a collection of symptoms and signs associated with a decrease in estrogen and other sex steroids involving changes to the labia majora/minora, clitoris, vestibule/introitus, vagina, urethra and bladder. The syndrome may include but is not limited to genital symptoms of dryness, burning and irritation; sexual symptoms of lack of lubrication, discomfort or pain and impaired function; and urinary symptoms of urgency, dysuria and recurrent urinary tract infections.

Cosmetic Surgery on the Clitoral Hood

Clitoral hood reduction, also known as *clitoral hoodectomy* or *clitoral unhooding*, involves surgically reducing the size of the clitoral hood and/or folds of skin that surround the clitoral glans by excising the skin.

Reasons

The goal of the surgery is to expose the clitoris in order to make it more aesthetically appealing and/or more sensitive for increased sexual pleasure. Women with purely aesthetic concerns may seek the surgery because they are concerned their clitoral hood is too large. Some women want to improve their self-esteem if they or their partner feel the folds of their clitoral hood are unsightly. Others may be concerned their clitoral hood looks larger or more prominent after having a labiaplasty. They may re-present for surgical correction to have their clitoral hood reduced with the purpose of restoring the aesthetic balance between their clitoral hood and their new labia minora.

Women with functional concerns may seek out this surgery to increase sexual pleasure for themselves and their sexual partner. Theoretically, it is believed that removing the clitoral hood exposes the clitoral glans, making it more sensitive, so the woman is better able to achieve orgasm through the thrusting movement of the penis during penetrative sex. However, no empirical studies to date support this notion.

Risks

Anecdotal evidence suggests that some women who have this surgery experience more sexual sensitivity while others experience sexual pain and anorgasmia (inability or difficulty reaching orgasm). The clitoral hood is continuous with the labia minora and is a specialised erogenous tissue in women which plays an important part in normal sexual functioning. Reducing clitoral hood tissue and exposing the clitoris, which are both rich in sensory nerves, is risky and care needs to be taken not to overexpose the glans of the clitoris. Removal of the clitoral hood may interfere with sexual pleasure by causing sexual pain and dissatisfaction. The procedure may impair sensual sensitivity and interfere with sexual arousal and the ability to achieve orgasm. Damage may result in chronic pain, such as clitorodynia and persistent genital arousal disorder, which are very difficult to treat. Other risks include dissatisfaction with the aesthetic result, infection, haematomas, abscess formation, phimosis (clitoral hood is fused over the glans of the clitoris), scarring, oedema, hypersensitivity, continuous pain and discomfort due to friction from clothes because the clitoris is over-exposed or there has been surgical damage to the glans or clitoral body due the removal of too much tissue.

Cosmetic Surgery on the Clitoral Glans

Clitoral repositioning, also known as *clitoroplasty*, involves surgically repositioning the tissues overlying the clitoral glans. The clitoris itself is not surgically operated on or repositioned.

Reasons

There is no literature on why women seek to undergo this procedure. The alleged purpose is to enhance the appearance or sexual functioning of the clitoris to increase sexual sensitivity and responsiveness.

Risks

As noted in relation to clitoral hood reduction surgery, there are a number of complications that may arise when exposing or repositioning the clitoris. Incisions can cause contractures or strangling of the clitoral tip causing *phimosis* whereby the clitoral hood is fused over the clitoris and cannot retract. The procedure runs a high risk of severing the vascular supply to the clitoris, causing haemorrhage and necrosis, clitoral pain and insensitivity. These risks are higher if the procedure is done simultaneously with other genital cosmetic surgical procedures.

Cosmetic Surgery on the Anterior Wall of the Vagina

Cosmetic surgery on the anterior wall of the vagina is termed *G-spot amplification* and involves injecting foreign material, such as dermal filler, hyaluronic acid or a collagen-based substance or autologous fat transfer, into a predetermined mystical G-spot site to increase the size of the area, or in the case of fat transfer, to create a bumpy irregularity. Another method involves a partial excision of the woman's *pubocervical fascia* (anterior vagina wall) which is harvested and the tissue transferred to the mystical G-spot site to create tension.

Reasons

Essentially, G-spot amplification is where the mystical G-spot receives a *fake-over*. Cosmetic surgeons who perform the procedure state that it will enhance or improve women's vaginal orgasm to boost sexual pleasure. The predetermined mystical G-spot is identified by the surgeon placing his finger inside the woman's vagina and wriggling and poking it around until the female patient says, *'That's the spot!'*

Risks

There is no scientific literature or clinical evidence on G-spot amplification to verify the effectiveness or safety of the procedure. There is a lack of scientific data on the safety and effectiveness of injecting foreign material into a woman's vagina. The surgery is potentially very harmful to women's health and wellbeing and women who have this procedure may experience a reduction in sexual sensation. Other risks include: *lack of therapeutic effect, hyaluronic acid pulmonary embolism, persistent abscess and open sores, erosion of the vaginal wall through open sores and scarring, post-operative bleeding, infection, hematoma, hypersensitivity, urethrovaginal fistulas and periurethral pseudocysts, urinary complications including urinary tract infections, urinary retention and urethral irritation, accelerated hyaluronan re-absorptions and allergic reactions such as swelling, itching or redness.*

Cosmetic Surgery on the Hymen/ Vaginal Corona

Hymen reconstruction, also known as *hymenoplasty* or *revirgination*, involves surgical reconstruction of the hymen to a *virginal* state to bleed at coitus. Essentially, it is a cosmetic procedure to create a fake hymen/vaginal corona. A number of hymen/vaginal corona reconstruction techniques exist. For instance, if remnants or tags of the woman's hymen exist and are adequate, they may be sutured together to reconstruct the hymen/vaginal corona. If there are inadequate hymenal remnants, a new hymen may be created by excising a small section of the skin from the woman's vaginal wall which is then tailored with sutures to the hymenal ring. Another technique involves narrowing the women's vaginal orifice (*introital vaginoplasty*) to increase the probability of tearing. Yet another technique involves suturing or inserting a gelatine capsule containing a substance designed to mimic blood into the vaginal wall. The expectation is that the capsule will burst during intercourse, providing evidence of the woman's virginity.

Reasons

Anecdotally, hymen reconstructions are on the rise in Australia. There are a variety of reasons why women seek the surgery to have a clean slate, including a woman who is wanting to become a nun and women who have been sexually active wanting to have the surgery before getting married as a way to present themselves as virgins to their husband-to-be. An intact hymen/vaginal corona is highly valued in some cultures and is erroneously thought to provide proof of a bride's virginity. Many women seek hymen reconstruction for this reason and often request a certificate of virginity following the surgery. Some women have reported having the surgery to ensure blood loss at coitus, sometimes in conjunction with vaginal tightening, to avoid suspicion that they had sexual intercourse prior to marriage. Japanese students who have been studying or holidaying in the USA have also reported having hymen reconstructions before returning home, as virginity is also highly valued in that culture. Australian and American women have reported having the procedure to *gift* their husbands a *virgin experience*. Meanwhile, women who have been sexually abused or raped have reported having the procedure to feel *whole* again.

Risks

Hymen reconstruction is highly controversial. There are numerous articles about the procedure, however to date, no rigorous scientific papers exist and there is no clinical standardisation of surgical techniques. Surgeons who perform the surgery face an ethical dilemma. If they perform the procedure, they are perpetrating the myth that an intact hymen is a sign of virginity. However, if they refuse, they may be putting women at grave risk of harm and exploitation by unscrupulous practitioners if the surgery was to go underground.

Women who have hymen reconstruction surgery face serious risks. Scarring from hymen reconstruction surgery may cause dyspareunia and women may experience obstetric difficulties with vaginal delivery. Other complications include *vaginismus*, *wound dehiscence* (*separations of the incisions*), *infections, fistulas, haemorrhaging* and *incontinence*. Moreover, there is no guarantee that bleeding upon penetration will occur, the stitches may fall out or be identified if the woman is forced to undergo an examination before getting married. In some cultures, women who fail the virgin test not only risk bringing shame to their family, but also divorce and, in extreme cases, they are murdered.

Pressure to Perform & Unhappy Asymmetry

The messages women receive about their vulvas are that something is defective and their sexual responsiveness is lacking. Labiaplasty has received the most notoriety in the research. It is unclear why women would prefer to have one type of genital cosmetic surgery over another. Women are not only worried about their genital appearance, as in the case of labiaplasty, but they are equally concerned about their sexual functioning, as in G-spot amplification and vaginal tightening.

The requests from women for G-spot amplification indicate they feel the pressure to perform sexually. Women are led to believe that having an enlarged G-spot will improve their sex life, resulting in more powerful orgasms and more heightened levels of sexual arousal; however, no empirical studies support these notions. Women who request this type of genital cosmetic surgery may lack knowledge about sexual health and sexual functioning. Furthermore, the G-spot amplification procedure (trademark G-Shot®) is also highly controversial and may result in women experiencing a reduction in sexual sensation as well as other health risks. The medical professionals who inject dermal filler or collagen into this area to supposedly increase the size and sensitivity of the G-spot have been accused of medical fraud by profiting from women's insecurities regarding their sexual functioning.

It is unclear why women who are dissatisfied with the tightness of their vagina would seek out cosmetic surgery on the vaginal opening. It may be due to genital anatomical incompatibility of the vagina and penis. During penile-vaginal intercourse the size (length and thickness) of the partner's penis is important for some women and not for others. Other women may experience lack of sexual satisfaction or enjoyment if their sexual partner's penis lacks in length and/or girth. This raises the concern that for some individuals there is a perceived *unhappy asymmetry* between men's and women's bodies.

G-spot amplification, cosmetic vaginal tightening and all the other genital cosmetic surgeries offered to women, is yet another reason for women to feel abnormal and sexually inadequate. To address this chasm of unhappiness more education regarding the issues for women is apparent.

Cosmetic Surgery Cowboys

Most cosmetic surgeries, including female genital cosmetic surgery, are carried out by surgeons in the private health sector in Australia. The industry is largely unregulated and unaudited. In this context, female genital cosmetic surgery is performed by a range of practitioners, including plastic surgeons, cosmetic doctors and gynaecologists. As mentioned previously, it is currently legal for doctors with a basic medical degree and no formal specialist surgical training to perform cosmetic surgery in Australia. This lack of regulation is problematic as it potentially puts women seeking genital cosmetic surgery at risk from *cowboy* practitioners who are not professionally trained.

A major misconception among the Australian public is that cosmetic surgery is safe and painless. However, it is important to recognise the inherent risks involved in undergoing these procedures. The number of episodes of harm to women are increasing in unregulated offices by practitioners who do not have the appropriate qualifications or training to perform the cosmetic procedures they are undertaking. Shocking practices are exposed in Australia's cosmetic surgery industry by Four Corners in a joint investigation with The Age and Sydney Morning Herald. **TRIGGER & CONTENT WARNING** to viewers this documentary shows alarming surgical practices, graphic scenes and nudity: *Cosmetic Cowboys: The unregulated world of cosmetic surgery.*

PORN TOWN

HIJACKING WOMEN'S SEXUALITY

There can be a number of influences which result in women developing genital image anxiety, including pornography. Pornography deserves more discussion as it can have a devastating effect on women's sexual self-esteem and sexuality. Pornography is hijacking the healthy sexual development of young women by setting the agenda for women's sexuality. Pornography is setting women up for failure through heartache and disappointment, as it rarely sets the tone for developing a healthy and happy relationship with your partner.

Over the decades I have spoken to hundreds of women of all ages and, to a lesser extent, men, whose sexual lives have been tarnished and even, in some instances, devastated by having pornography in their lives. As a psychologist, to university students, I have counselled many young women who are hooking up with males who have been conditioned erotically through pornography and how this porn script is creating problems with their relationship and sexual self-esteem. I have seen first-hand how pornography is crushing women's spirit. Men are not immune and often tell me they wish they were never introduced to pornography. Some men I have counselled who use pornography experience poor mental health, erectile problems, loss of employment, blackmail, financial problems and the breakdown of their marriage or relationship. Men's sexuality has equally been hijacked by pornography and promotes toxic masculinity.

If your first contact with sex is via mainstream pornography, this can be a concern for the healthy development of your attitudes towards sex and relationships. Extreme sex sells – if it was just *vanilla* normal sex, people would not watch mainstream pornography. *Porn Town* is where women are dehumanised and if you think about it, it also dehumanises men. Pornography is not sex education. Well, it might teach you the mechanics but will not teach you about intimacy. It teaches men that women are just holes for men to put things in. Mainstream pornography presents a warped view of what healthy sex is not about. Mainstream pornography is about what is hot for men and often depicts men humiliating and degrading women. Acceptance of pornography varies between women and men. In the context of a relationship many couples debate whether pornography is to be accepted, tolerated or condemned.

Hardcore porn that depicts violence and choking is normalised through porn. There is no excuse for violence against women. Sex should be in a safe and consensual way. Porn Town is detrimental not only to women, but to men too. Men may struggle with relationships and experience erectile difficulties. Men who live in Porn Town have been conditioned erotically and have expectations of what they can do to a woman's body. They are also conditioned erotically to have expectations of what a woman's body should look like – for instance, large breasts, no pubic hair and no labia minora. They may also harbour unrealistic expectations about sex, which in Porn Town is all about performance. For instance, they may believe that their penis should stay hard for hours – just like they have seen in Porn Town. Some men also believe that the sex acts they see in Porn Town are normal. Males are watching porn from a young age and they are not literate about what a healthy and normal relationship looks like. Porn Town is where you learn about sex that is not considered to be healthy in the real-world. Many young women are growing up with young men who have been porn conditioned. This is very concerning as more young women are learning about sex and relationships through Porn Town.

The script of sex in pornography is performative and not real – it's a fantasy, like Hollywood sex but on steroids. You won't get the facts about sex and relationships on your visit to Porn Town. It's easy to watch porn – it is more difficult to have a healthy relationship. If porn is your sex education, it is most certainly not going to teach you about women's sexual pleasure or how to build a real connection with a woman. When you watch mainstream pornography there is no such thing as *consent*. The sex depicted in pornography is rough and violent, only prioritising male pleasure. Female pleasure does not exist in Porn Town.

Globally, more women are viewing mainstream pornography, with hardcore pornography becoming more mainstream as well. A lot of more global porn traffic for both men and women occurred throughout the COVID-19 pandemic, due to the social isolation of lockdowns and quarantine. However, for women who are dissatisfied by mainstream pornography, prefer to subscribe to *ethical porn*, sometimes referred to as *feminist porn* or *fair-trade porn*. In response, more women are turning to *ethical porn* in which sexual relationships are not portrayed as misogynistic. Ethical porn centres of depictions of women's pleasure, healthy relationships and non-violent sexual behaviours. Ethical porn is shot from a woman's gaze, involving consensual relationships and more realistic sex. The performers in these films are paid fairly for their work and have safe working conditions which does not occur in mainstream pornography.

Many health professionals are concerned about the trends in pornography exposure and how it affects the sexual socialisation of young men and young women. Pornography misinforms young people and their understanding of which sexual behaviours are acceptable or rewarding. So many people are watching porn and having sex, yet it is still difficult for people to ask for help regarding their relationship or sexual problems.

Pornography offers an avenue for you to explore your own sexuality. However, many of the behaviours and sexual acts that are performed in pornography are not considered by mainstream society to be normative or enjoyable. Researchers and health professionals are concerned about the negative impact that pornography has on young women's (and young men's) sexual health and mental health. For example, some young heterosexual men are incorporating sexual behaviours, such as anal sex, that they see in pornography into their real relationships. Many young women are aware that their male peers are looking at porn where anal sex is commonly depicted. These young women say that their boyfriends will ask and pressure them to have anal sex. Women report that they feel they are competing with porn sex – and this can cause issues within their relationships.

Violence against women is *NOT* sexy. Nothing is wrong with you if you say no to sex or other sexual activities:

- It is okay to say *NO* to having vaginal sex with your sexual partner.
- It is okay to say *NO* to having anal sex with your sexual partner.
- It is okay to say *NO* to having your hair pulled by your sexual partner.
- It is okay to say *NO* to being hit by your sexual partner.
- It is okay to say *NO* to being choked by your sexual partner.

- It is okay to say *NO* to being pinched by your sexual partner.
- It is okay to say *NO* to being punched/slapped/spat on/urinated on by your sexual partner.
- It is okay to say *NO* to watching pornography with your sexual partner.

Relationship review – Here are a few questions for you to ponder about the effect porn may have had on your sexuality:

- What has been your sexual journey?
- How has pornography shaped your sexual self?
- Is your sexual script about making sure your male partner is satisfied?
- Is your sexual partner's sexual script about getting their sexual needs met?

Congratulations, *Vulva Image Warrior!* This is the end of this section of your journey to becoming an expert about your own sexuality, or, as I like to also call it, achieving *labia liberation*. Next on your *Vulva Image Warrior* journey is exploring how to increase your genital image confidence. You will also discover how to have a *voluptuous vulva* through strategies such as mindfulness to address any genital image troubles and anxieties you may be experiencing.

V-SECTION FOUR

Vulva Victory

We cannot directly affect the images, we can drain them of their power. We can turn away from them, look directly at one another, . . .
We can lift ourselves and other women out of the myth.
– Naomi Wolf

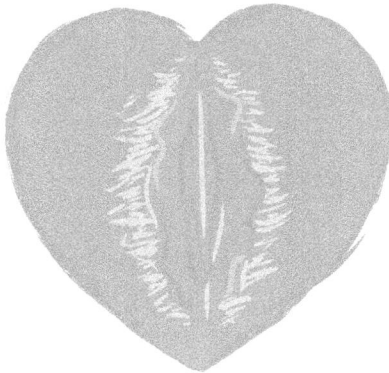

Beyond the Birds and the Bees

How to Have a Chat to a Health Professional About Your Vulva

Many women request some sort of female genital cosmetic surgery without being medically or psychologically assessed beforehand as to the suitability of undergoing such a procedure. It is important to explore your motivations for seeking it out. Not an easy thing to do. It can be challenging to come to terms with feelings and thoughts you may be having about your genitals. It is important to talk it out with your trusted doctor. You could just say, '*Hi, I am worried and was wondering if I look normal down there,*' or, '*I am worried that my labia minora does not look normal.*' It is concerning for many doctors that some women will avoid or delay having a pap smear due to feeling their genitals are abnormal. Doctors who work in women's health will be familiar with the issues concerning genital image anxiety.

If you are considering having female genital cosmetic surgery, know that this is a big decision. It is important that you are sure this is the right decision for you. In some cases, female genital cosmetic surgery can resolve an issue that is causing you concern and it may even alleviate your distress. However, for others, female genital cosmetic surgery is a symptom of a deep-seated psychological issue. In these instances, the cosmetic surgery is likely not to solve your issue and may make things worse. Sure, you may look different down there after the surgery, but it is quite likely that your distress or underlying issues will remain the same. Cosmetic surgery on your genitals may not transform your life and your concerns may be better met by talking to your doctor and/ or psychologist.

Nip it in the bud! It's important to put an end to any worries you may have about your body before the problem worsens. The sooner you talk about your fears and anxieties the better it will be for you. Doctors have seen a lot of vulvas and therefore have seen a lot of diversity in women's genitalia. This is very reassuring to know. They are without a doubt the right person to go to with your genital image concerns. It might be helpful to make an extended appointment with your doctor so you both have the time to talk about your concerns. Your doctor will probably ask you questions, such as, '*In what way are you unhappy about how your genitals look?*' It is important to build a relationship with your general practitioner as it helps them understand your feelings and for you to build rapport and trust with them. Everyone's situation is unique.

At your consultation, you can expect the following:

- The doctor might ask you if you would like to have a physical examination.

- Your doctor will provide you with some practical solutions if you are experiencing labia discomfort.

- It might be necessary for your doctor to refer you to see a specialist adolescent and paediatric gynaecologist.

- Your doctor may offer to refer you to a mental health professional to support you.

- If your doctor has identified that you have body dysmorphic disorder, they will offer to refer you to see a psychologist or a psychiatrist for a thorough assessment and diagnosis.

Here are some questions that your doctor may ask you that will assist them in understanding your situation:

- What type of exercise do you do?
- What sort of clothing do you wear?
- When did the irritation start?
- Do you remove your pubic hair?
- Do you have sexual intercourse?
- Is there discomfort or pain when you have sex?
- How is your genital image anxiety affecting your life/your relationships?
- What do you know about the function of your vulva?
- Have you been bullied or teased about the appearance of your genitals?

To help start the conversation with your doctor or health professional, take a copy of *The Happy Vulva* with you to your appointment. You can rehearse what you are going to say or give your doctor a note indicating your concern. For example:

Dear Doctor

This note is to help me talk to you about a problem I am worried about. I have been reading The Happy Vulva and have a copy to show you. The issue I would like to explore with you is on page ...

Thanks for your time and understanding.

You may have more than one concern affecting your genital image self-esteem. You can write down your concerns which can be a helpful guide for when you go to the appointment.

Here are some other questions for you to consider that may be contributing to your genital image anxiety.

Do you feel pressured to change because of someone else?

It is very understandable that you would want to please your partner. However, if you change your genital appearance this may not actually change the relationship.

It is important to ask yourself:

- What is it actually saying about my partner?
- Has my partner accepted the real me?
- Where do they get their values from?
- Is my partner gaslighting me about my body and sex?

Gaslighting is insidious, so it is not always obviously detectable. It is a form of emotional abuse designed to convince you that something is wrong with you. It can affect all areas of your life. In the bedroom your male sexual partner may say you are not sexual enough or that your genitals look wrong. Some women have told me that their male sexual partner will withhold intimacy until they remove all their pubic hair. Women find this very confronting as they feel their male sexual partner wants them to have a pubis that looks like a pre-pubescent girl. This is particularly troubling for those women who are mothers of young girls. It is also distressing for women who have been sexually abused as a child. These attitudes deny you the ability to make decisions about your own sexuality. Women find it hard to say no to their sexual partner as they want to please them and see it as their responsibility for keeping the sexual flames glowing in the relationship, rather than being mutual in the context of a healthy relationship. It decreases women's ability to connect and get help from others because of the confusion and shame attached. If you are experiencing any distress or concerns, please don't hesitate to seek out professional support.

Some women who experiment by completely denuding their mons pubis find it very exciting. For other women, this can be confronting. My friends who are now grandmothers have said to me that we need a campaign to 'bring back the bush'. They are concerned that their granddaughters will see that their mother has no pubic hair, but Nana or Nonna does. These grandmothers have said they are worried that this will cause confusion for young girls (and boys). Many young men have not seen a woman with pubic hair. What happens if the fashion changes where pubic hair makes a comeback and it becomes de rigueur to have hair down there? If a hairy pubis becomes fashionable again then this will be challenging for women who have lasered away every skerrick of pubic hair. They won't be able to pivot to the new trend. Perhaps we will see the sale of merkins (pubic hair wigs) skyrocket!

Should I get counselling before female genital cosmetic surgery?

If your motivation is that you feel that female genital cosmetic surgery will make you feel normal, then you may need to consider counselling, or at the very least discuss it over with your doctor. Remember, that there is absolutely nothing wrong with wanting to take care of your appearance. However, by having some type of female genital *cosmetic* surgery may not make you feel normal down there.

FGCS?
ASK YOURSELF THESE
FIVE QUESTIONS

- Do you have a serious belief that you are deformed in some way and that genital cosmetic surgery is the only answer to making you feel normal?

- Are you having the genital cosmetic surgery because you see this as a way of correcting a deep personal or perceived flaw in yourself?

- When you think about that perceived flaw, do you feel shame?

- When you think about that perceived flaw, is it affecting your self-esteem?

- Do you feel that no one will love you or accept the way you are unless you change the appearance of your vulva?

Do You See Female Genital Cosmetic Surgery as Problem-Solving?

Cosmetic surgery of any kind is a radical problem-solving technique that may have negative consequences. Don't believe all the hype that some of the cosmetic surgery clinics espouse about having your labia minora amputated or burnt off. No type of cosmetic surgery can guarantee to fix your relationship issues or low self-esteem. You may recover from the cosmetic surgery and end up feeling the same person you were pre-surgery.

One of the motivations of writing this book is the many disturbing stories that I and many of my colleagues have heard in this space. The main theme women disclose is had they been made aware of the issues pre-surgery they may not have gone ahead. They often feel duped by the cosmetic surgeon for not informing them their labia minora is of normal appearance.

After you have considered all the issues and you have decided that female genital cosmetic surgery would enhance your life, then this is fantastic for you. My job is done – you are more aware of the issues and you feel this puts you in a position to make a more informed choice of whether to proceed with a procedure (or not).

Patching Up Your Genitals May Not Patch Up Your Problems

Some women carry a burden with them that they are too embarrassed to discuss their feelings about spending time and money on such a private area of their body. However, when you are ready it would be very beneficial if you could reach out to someone you trust about your feelings. I recommend you make an appointment with a qualified psychologist. Talking about your feelings may be a more worthwhile investment than having potentially risky and unnecessary female genital cosmetic surgery. Many women have been alone in dealing with these issues. You will probably find it very helpful to have a discussion with someone who is empathic and sensitive to your feelings, past hurts and fears.

You can never stop learning about sex. However, finding information on sex by scrolling through Google, YouTube or mainstream pornography sites are not the best sex education tools around. Google and YouTube can have some helpful information but will not replace information provided by a qualified and experienced health professional. It's a bit like consulting Dr Google first about a health issue (we've all done that!) rather than making an appointment with your general practitioner. It seems we are all self-diagnosing these days and problem solving using the internet. Essentially, we are putting off dealing with a sexual concern or health problem. Delaying getting evidence-based information about anxieties about sex can be problematic and not solve the issue at all – it might even make it worse. You can talk about your concern with a qualified health professional.

Genital & Body Image Acceptance

Stop It! No More Body Trash Talk

The way many parents are trying to build their daughters' body confidence is by telling them that they are beautiful *all the time*. This does not build body confidence. Constantly telling someone they are beautiful sends the message that beauty and appearance are the most important things about them. The biggest winners in the beauty games are indubitably the cosmetic surgeons who can cut us up, the beauticians who inject us with dermal fillers and the companies that sell us weight loss products. These multinational industries thrive on women not having body self-confidence.

Constantly telling your daughter that she is beautiful, that her beauty and appearance is what defines her, is only setting her up for failure. Being *beautiful* becomes the thing they believe that defines them. Young girls are growing up with messages not only from the media but from their mothers, aunts and grandmothers – who for decades have been fed a diet of body hatred from the media. Young girls don't need to be on social media to learn about body hatred. They are absorbing the body hating messages from an early age from the women around them.

What we need to do is to stop talking and listening to the language of body hatred. As women, we need to stop talking about other women's bodies, who has gained weight, who looks hot and who does not look hot. As adult women we need to start talking about other things with girls and young women such as politics, agriculture, health, technology, world peace, medicine, art, leadership, fun, the environment, sport, adventures, theatre, engineering, mathematics, further education, stock market, real-estate, science, biology, physics, comedy, school, sport, friends and music. I think you get the picture – to talk about anything but diet and appearance. Discuss with your daughter and young girls in your life other things that stimulate and occupy their minds, instead of funnelling them into thinking and feeling that the only thing they need to be good at is being *beautiful* and *hot*. If you have a young girl in your life, it would be good to discuss age-appropriate information about how her body functions and about healthy relationships.

As women, we too often defer to men for information about our sexuality. However, it is more likely that you know more about your body than your male partner or peers. It is inevitable that many men have learnt about the female body by fumbling around in the dark or via the internet. If I sound harsh, I make no apologies. Men too, have had poor sexual education and many turn to porn as their sex coach. Porn just makes men ignorant of women's sexual needs and therefore uninterested in exploring them. Porn harms men too. Some men struggle to maintain a healthy relationship and others can experience sexual dysfunction. I have heard firsthand from women of all ages about the sexual ineptitude of their partners. We need to stop protecting fragile egos and succumbing to sexual proclivities that we do not find enjoyable. Young women tell me they worry they are *asexual* because they don't feel sexual desire or sexually aroused. Many say their male sexual partner will hop on top of her and pound away and after climaxing asks if his performance was good. This sounds very unsatisfying – why bother, girls? Many tell me that men pester them to have anal sex telling them that it is normal and every girl is doing it. I am here to tell you that not every female is having or desiring anal sex and, FYI, many women also don't like to be choked. This is the sexual script of porn sex. Women need to stop blaming themselves about the bad sex they are having. It is clear to me why so many women are confused about their sexuality.

As women, we are focussed on pleasing our partners to maintain the relationship. We can better inform ourselves and those men who are important in our lives, about bedroom matters and manners. Many men would say they wish their female partner would tell them what they like to happen and how they can please them. Unfortunately, and paradoxically, due to living in a hypersexualised society, women's bodies have been a mystery to themselves. The remedy to this knowledge gap is to employ an inquiring mind and to search out appropriate information that will guide you in building your sexual confidence. Another way is to seek out like-minded women with whom you can talk about such things.

Body Image
in the Bedroom

How women feel about their body and their genitals can affect their sexual experience. The worries or distractions about genital appearance interfere with women's ability to remain erotically focused during sexual activity. Researchers who have explored women's body and genital image self-consciousness in the sexual setting have found women who were more self-conscious about their body and genitals during sexual activity report several difficulties. They experience poor genital image and genital self-image, poor sexual self-esteem, low levels of sexual pleasure, lower levels of desire to have sex, difficulties with sexual arousal, inability and difficulties having an orgasm and more sexual pain or discomfort during sexual activity. Women who are self-conscious during sexual activity will avoid some sexual practices such as oral sex and masturbation.

Women who have positive genital image are more likely to engage in more frequent sexual activities, such as foreplay, intercourse, oral sex, masturbation and vibrator use. They also experience more orgasms and are more likely to have regular gynaecological exams to keep their sexual health in check. Research sometimes just tells us what we already intuitively know – that if we don't think and feel good about ourselves that this can translate into having difficulties in the bedroom. A woman who has positive feelings about her genitalia and about exposing her body and genitals in sexual settings is less likely to be distracted by negative feelings such as self-consciousness. They also are less likely to feel embarrassment, shame or anxiety towards the appearance of her genitals and body and more likely to feel sexual desire.

The following pages will discuss strategies about how to be more positive about your genital image and less self-conscious about your body and genitals in the bedroom.

Dancing Fairy In Your Undies

How to Enhance your Sexual Vibe

In my late teens and early twenties, my good girlfriend, Carolina, and I would talk all things and more about our sex lives. We covered all sorts of topics from masturbation and the pill to sex. Carolina called the feeling of being turned on as *having a dancing fairy in her undies* – which I thought was funny, curious and intriguing all at the same time. Other girlfriends of the day would call the feeling of sexual desire and arousal as *getting wet* or feeling *horny, randy* or *hot*. I much prefer the term *dancing fairies in your undies* to describe this awesome sexual feeling.

Dancing Vulva Fairy is a euphemism which refers to feeling sexual pleasure or feeling *turned on*. This sexual pleasure is centered in your genitals and then spreads throughout your body. Sexual pleasure are intense feelings of pleasure caused by sexual triggers and can cause changes in your body. Sexual pleasure feelings also cause changes in your thoughts and emotions. *Dancing Vulva Fairies* need good enough, or near good enough, conditions to enhance sexual feelings, sexual thoughts and sexual emotions.

Your *Dancing Vulva Fairy* is your inner coach. Learning about the power of your *Dancing Vulva Fairy* will help you maintain erotic focus. Your *Nasty Vulva Pixie* is the inner sprite that prevents you from feeling sexual pleasure or feeling *turned* on. Your *Nasty Vulva Pixie* is the arched nemesis of your *Dancing Vulva* Fairy. It is important to recognise how your *Nasty Vulva Pixie* operates and what to do when this nasty little sprite activates your genital image anxieties. Genital image anxieties come in the form of automatic negative thoughts that affect your self-esteem and distract you from feeling positive sexual thoughts and feelings. Recognising your automatic negative thoughts will help you to identify how your *Nasty Vulva Pixie* style of thinking contributes to your genital image anxiety. Identifying your unhelpful thinking can help guide you to make positive changes. It is important to catch yourself when you engage in negative thinking. For instance, there may be certain situations that activate your automatic negative thoughts, or maybe they are just fleeting thoughts that pop into your mind. For the following exercises you need to bring out your best detective skills.

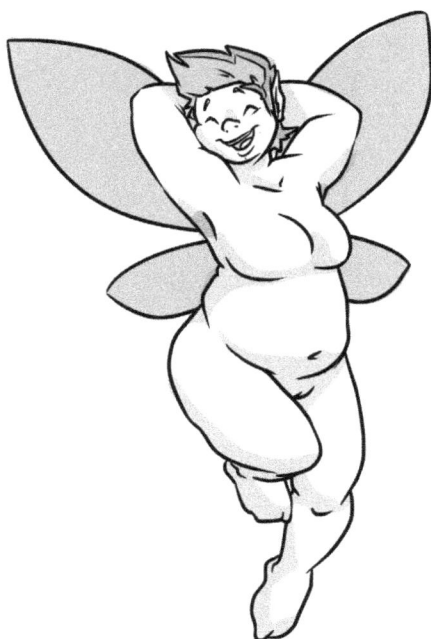

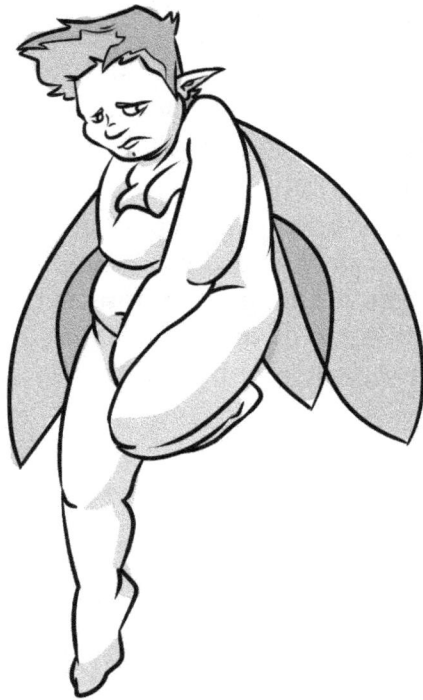

LEARNING TO SAY YES TO YOUR DANCING VULVA FAIRY

The following visualisation exercise is helpful in assisting you to catch and wrangle your automatic negative thoughts.

Picture this: sitting on one shoulder you have a *Nasty Vulva Pixie* representing your inner critic. The *Nasty Vulva Pixie* is busy saying all sorts of things which make you feel self-conscious, worried and more anxious about your genitals. The negative energy that exudes from the *Nasty Vulva Pixie* makes you tense, and this distraction stops you from focusing on sexual pleasure and further erodes your sexual self-esteem.

Now imagine sitting on your other shoulder is the *Dancing Vulva Fairy*, and she represents your positive inner coach. Your *Dancing Vulva Fairy* is there to help you relax and focus on sexual pleasure. Your *Dancing Vulva Fairy* is tired of being drowned out and dominated by the *Nasty Vulva Pixie*. The good news is that your *Dancing Vulva Fairy* can stop the *Nasty Vulva Pixie* having their wicked and evil way with you.

Learning how to drown out the noise and negativity of the *Nasty Vulva Pixie* is an important first step to help increase your sexual self-esteem. To help make all your genital anxieties dissipate, it is important to highlight the positive voice of your *Dancing Vulva Fairy*. In doing so you will be better able to focus on sexual pleasure and focus on sexual sensation.

We all have moments when we listen to our inner critic. The goal of this exercise is for you to learn to be able to catch and recognise that the *Nasty Vulva Pixie* is the voice of your genital anxiety. This exercise is to make you more aware of your negative thinking style and using distraction and counterstatements to wrangle that *Nasty Vulva Pixie* and put her in her place. This will increase your sexual self-esteem so you feel more confident about yourself. It won't happen overnight and will take some practice to be able to harness your genital anxieties. It is important to remember these habits can at least be diluted, if not completely broken. The following exercise was adapted from Dr Rosie King's (2004) patient handout, *Declare war on automatic negative thoughts!*

Vote No to Your Nasty Vulva Pixie

As part of your personal campaign to manage your genital image anxiety, it is important to write down your automatic negative thoughts. This is detective time – we need to know exactly what sort of negative *Nasty Vulva Pixie* thoughts you are dealing with. This is not always an easy thing to do as those thoughts can happen so quickly that you hardly even notice them. However, the very act of outing *Nasty Vulva* Pixie dilutes her power.

For example:

> *What if my boyfriend wants to have sex and notices something wrong with my genitals?*

Below is a list of things you can do when you catch yourself thinking negatively about your sexual self by using these inner coach strategies. It is a good idea to choose one or two of these suggestions. You may notice that one of the strategies you use has a stronger impact than another strategy. You may also notice that your inner critic aka *Nasty Vulva Pixie* is sometimes louder and more persistent at certain times. This is all good detective work you are doing. By figuring out what works and what does not work for you, is all important in learning ways to manage your genital image anxiety. Your inner coach will be guiding your positive *Dancing Vulva Fairy* by reminding you to keep going and to try one more time.

When you catch yourself worrying about genital anxieties before a sexual situation

Choose one or two of the following *Vulva Mantras* to bring out your *Dancing Vulva Fairy*:

All I have to do is focus on sensation.

All I have to do is focus on pleasure.

All I have to do is focus on the feelings.

All I have to do is focus on sight/sound/smell/taste/touch.

It is important for you to repeat these statements over and over as this achieves these three important outcomes:

- Helps you to block out the automatic negative thoughts of the *Nasty Vulva Pixie*.
- Helps you to refocus on pleasure and sensation so you can be erotically focused.
- Creates space for you to enhance your good conditions to enjoy the sexual activity you are having, desiring or wanting to have.

When you catch yourself worrying about genital anxieties during a sexual situation

When you catch your *Nasty Vulva Pixie* causing you to worry about your genital image during a sexual situation, you can choose one or two of the following *Vulva Mantras* to bring out your *Dancing Vulva Fairy*:

This thinking is not helpful.

All I need to do is to be in the moment.

I am focusing on how my body feels.

I am focusing on pleasurable sensations and on (the name of your sexual partner).

If you notice that your mind wanders to the negative thinking patterns of the *Nasty Vulva Pixie*, choose to say instead:

Come on mind, let's get back to the moment, get back to pleasure and to sensation, back to the Dancing Vulva Fairies.

Whatever that Nasty Vulva Pixie thought is, I don't need to follow it now – all I have to do is focus on pleasure and sensation.

When you catch yourself worrying about genital anxieties outside a sexual situation

You could say to your *Nasty Vulva Pixie*:

I am not going to let myself think like this. This thinking is not helpful.

I am going to think about how cool it feels.

You can also change the pattern by not only noticing your inner critic and using coping statements or counterstatements, but also doing something physical to help disengage from your automatic negative self-talk. Using distraction in a physical way is a great technique in helping you ignore your *Nasty Vulva Pixie*. For example, when you are driving and you notice your *Nasty Vulva Pixie* has popped into your thoughts, try turning the music up or change the song or radio station. You could wind the window down to get a burst of fresh air to distract you. If you are sitting on the couch and the negative genital self-talk begins, get up. If you are daydreaming, move around and do something else. When you change your pattern of behaviour also say a counterstatement with energy and increased intensity, it can also give your *Nasty Vulva Pixie* thoughts the message that you mean business! For instance:

> *Stop! That is anxiety and not helpful and I don't let myself think that anymore!*

The more skills and strategies, the better equipped you will be to manage your negative genital image self-talk and be able to hear your *Dancing Vulva Fairy*.

Catastrophising is a type of negative self-talk that makes you feel more anxious and will sabotage your ability to get sexually aroused. It is also called *awfulising* – where you view your situation as terrible, awful, dreadful and horrible.

> *What if my partner gets annoyed with me if I can't relax? I will lose this relationship.*

Instead of the above automatic negative thought you could substitute a more optimistic and realistic coping statement:

> *Yes, I am worried my partner will be disappointed if we don't have oral sex but we can still enjoy making love.*

Alternatively, you can turn the following *Nasty Vulva Pixie* statement from:

What will my genitals look like during oral sex?

To a statement that represents a plan for change and encourages your *Dancing Vulva Fairy* to come out and get more enjoyment by saying:

I am going to focus on how my body feels during oral sex or when we make love.

Singing and silly voices – Another great technique is to sing silently in your head any of the *Nasty Vulva Pixie* statements to the tune of *Twinkle, twinkle little star* in a high-pitched pixie voice.

You could practice these exercises while you engage in self-love through masturbation. This will get you used to focusing on body sensations and not cognitive interruptions (aka *Nasty Vulva Pixie* thoughts) in preparation for sexual activity with your partner.

Over-predictions and jumping to conclusions can cause a great deal of emotional distress. Changing the pattern or managing your automatic negative thoughts can be a challenge. It can be very helpful to speak with a psychologist or sex-therapist who has experience with cognitive and behaviour or allied therapies. What we think (cognitions) and what we do (behaviours) have a profound effect on the way we feel. A qualified and experienced therapist will work with you on formulating strategies in a safe and confidential environment.

Vulva Mindfulness & Vulva Guided Imagery

Learning How to Focus on Your Body & Sensations to Increase Sexual Arousal & Experience Genital Pleasure

The following exercises will help you maintain a sex-positive lens and discover or rediscover your sexual appetite.

Cognitive distractions (aka the *Nasty Vulva Pixie* thoughts) majorly inhibit women's ability to become and remain sexually aroused during sexual activity. The practice of mindfulness-based meditation has been found to improve women's sexual desire and increase their arousal both mentally and physically (lubrication), which in turn increases their ability to achieve orgasm, reduce sexual pain and to overall improve women's experience of sexual satisfaction.

It is recommended that you speak with your doctor if you continue to experience pain during sex.

I recommend to women that they complete a basic mindfulness course prior to starting this exercise. It has been shown women who have engaged in regular mindfulness practice are able to feel more aroused, more quickly. Other potential benefits of mindfulness-based meditation include reduction of negative body image and negative genital image, reduction around feelings of low self-esteem, reduction of depression and anxiety, reduction of chronic pain and improvement in sleep quality. Mindfulness-based meditation is defined as having *non-judgemental present moment awareness* – to be in the here and now and to focus on one point in time. With practice, you can re-train your brain and be able to let all the *Nasty Vulva Pixie* thoughts go away.

CONTRAINDICATIONS & CAVEATS TO USING MINDFULNESS

Mindfulness may temporarily exacerbate symptoms of anxiety. When this happens it could be a side effect of becoming more aware of your physical sensations; a mild, fleeting discomfort that may quickly pass particularly as you become more adept. If you experience traumatic memories or you sense panic or distress, it is important to stop and take a break from the practice. If discomfort continues, please seek psychological support and/or complete a mindfulness program with a qualified health professional.

In fact, I strongly suggest to those who have experienced sexual trauma to complete an eight-week program with a mental health professional with expertise in trauma. It is important as mindfulness may allow traumatic memories to come to the forefront of our consciousness. This is particularly true when we are practicing mindfulness on the body areas which were the focus of abuse. However, with the appropriate support, general mindfulness and vulva focused mindfulness can assist us to process the trauma and transcend symptoms. It can also dissipate any criticism of our body parts we have experienced from abusers.

Tuning-In To Your Body & Brain in Three Steps

The intention of the *Vulva & Body Scan* exercise is to create a positive mindset to give you the optimum chance to feel passion and pleasure. The purpose of the *Vulva & Body Scan* is for you to tune in to your body, including your genitals, to reconnect to your physical self and notice any sensations you are feeling without judgement.

During the *Vulva & Body Scan* you will focus on and explore each region of your body. The theme of the *Vulva & Body Scan* is to lightly check in to see what is present in each body region and notice the sensations, temperature, there may be tingling or there may be nothing at all. With consistent practice most people become aware of a cacophony of sensations. What is important now is the act of paying attention. What you sense is not as important as the act of paying attention. The act of paying attention strengthens the brain and its capacity to focus, thereby ultimately increasing your sensual perceptions. As you notice your mind wandering away from your awareness of your body in the present and into daydreams of the past or future, just reconnect and guide your mind back to the part of the body you were exploring.

It is important to practice the *Vulva & Body Scan* twice a day for one week in preparation before moving onto the *Vulva Mindfulness* and *Vulva Guided Imagery* exercises.

This activity is important to check in with yourself on what is pleasant to you. Our minds are prone to distraction or wandering – even at the best of times. Train the brain to be present, fully attentive and in the moment, to feel at ease and without distraction. These qualities will help you be less self-conscious about your body during sex. Some women tell me they like to practice the *Vulva & Body Scan* exercise when lying in bed before they go to sleep and/or when they wake up. What a great way to start and end the day!

The *Vulva Guided Imagery* exercise is a mind-body intervention which evokes and generates mental images that re-create your sensory perceptions of sights, sounds, smells, tastes and touch. *Vulva Guided Imagery* is a method of relaxation which concentrates your mind on positive images to reduce feelings of genital image anxiety. This exercise was adapted from psychotherapist, Diane Ervine's 2009 workshop: *Working with Women's Sexual Concerns.*

With practice using the *Vulva Mindfulness* and *Vulva Guided Imagery* exercises you may notice that you are better able to experience sexual interest, desire and arousal. You may also notice with all this sexual excitement that you experience more sexual satisfaction. Expect to also experience pleasure and sensations in your genitals such as warmth, tingling and/or throbbing.

The practice of *Vulva Mindfulness* and *Vulva Guided Imagery* will help you learn to be less judgemental and more accepting of yourself. An added benefit of the practice of *Vulva Mindfulness* and *Vulva Guided Imagery* is that you will find yourself to be less judgemental and more accepting of your partner. The *Vulva Mindfulness* and *Vulva Guided Imagery* exercises will help foster and build intimacy, so you will experience a deeper connection with your partner. Women who are mindful during sex are paying close attention to the sensations of their partners touch or the sounds of their partner's breathing. Learning to stay mindful will help keep your mind off distractions getting in the way of you having satisfying sex.

STEP 1
THE VULVA & BODY SCAN EXERCISE

It is important to do this first exercise twice a day for one week as preparation before moving on to the *Vulva Mindfulness* and *Vulva Guided Imagery* exercises. At every step *focus on the slow flow of your breath rising and falling*:

- Sit in a chair in a comfortable position, allowing your head to float lightly upwards and your eyes closed gently. The intention of this practice is to cultivate your attention so that you are alert but relaxed.
- Take a few moments to get in touch with the movement of your breath and the sensations you feel in your body. Check out of your thinking and busy mind to arrive with attention and the mindfulness that your body is at rest now.
- Bring your awareness to the physical sensations in your body, especially to the sensations of touch or pressure where your body makes contact with the chair.
- On each out-breath allow yourself to let go and to sink a little deeper into the chair.

- Move your attention to the whole of your left leg, experiencing a letting go with the out-breath of the whole of your left leg.
- Move your attention to the whole of your right leg, experiencing a letting go with the out-breath of the whole of your right leg.
- Move your attention and breathing into the whole of your genitals, then to your vulva and vagina.
- Move your attention to the pelvis – the whole of your pelvis, top and bottom, hip-to-hip, moving up to your abdomen, the small of your back your upper back and chest and breasts.
- Become aware and breathing into the whole of your left arm, allowing tension to release as you breathe out.
- Become aware and breathing into the whole of your right arm, allowing tension to release as you breathe out.
- Become aware of and breathing into your neck and shoulders, allowing tension to release as you breathe out.
- Become aware of the whole of your head, breathing into and allowing a release from the whole of your head.
- Become aware of your head, neck and shoulders. right arm, left arm, breasts, chest and back, stomach, small of the back, pelvis, genitals, right leg and left leg.
- Now slowly reverse the *Vulva & Body Scan* back down your body and repeat the scan as many times as you would like.
- Or become aware of your whole body and take a breath and slowly open your eyes.

You can also practice the *Vulva & Body Scan* exercise by listening to the audio by scanning the QR code at the back of this book.

STEP 2

VULVA MINDFULNESS-BASED EXERCISE

Setting the scene:

Have a piece of fruit or chocolate sitting on a plate beside you. It may also be handy to have a serviette to catch the juices of your delicious fruit or crumbs of creamy chocolate.

- Make sure you are sitting or lying comfortably allowing your body to feel relaxed.
- Pick up the piece of delicious fruit or creamy chocolate in your hand.

Now we will start with the *Vulva Mindfulness* exercise, at every step *focus on the slow flow of your breath rising and falling*:

- As you are sitting or lying comfortably, now, notice the sounds outside the room.
- Then notice the sounds inside the room.
- Gradually bring your awareness to your breath.
- Take a few moments of just breathing.
- Notice how it feels to be allowing your body to feel relaxed.

- Bring your attention to the delicious fruit or creamy chocolate in your hand.
- Notice the weight of how it feels in your hand.
- Notice if you have any urges to gobble up this delicious morsel.
- Bring your attention back to the sensation of the luscious treat in your hand.
- If your eyes are closed, gently open them, then look at the delicious juicy or creamy morsel in your hand.
- Observe its size, shape and colour and observe any responses (thoughts or sensations) you have towards it.
- Ever so slowly and gently bring the delicious juicy or creamy morsel to your nose and gently and slowly breath in its heavenly scent.
- Just for a moment or two appreciate the aroma.
- Notice if the urge to gobble up this delicious morsel may be even greater now (*noticing the slow flow of your breath rising and falling*).

Your goal is to simply be immersed in and simply focus on your experience... All you have to do is notice these things and enjoy the feeling of sitting or lying comfortably as you take in the aroma of the delicious juicy or creamy morsel.

Now you are ready to move on to Step 3: *The Vulva Guided Imagery Exercise.*

Step 3
The Vulva Guided Imagery Exercise

We use the *Vulva Mindfulness* exercise to lead you into the *Vulva Guided Imagery* exercise to help you relax more and more. At every step, *focus on the slow flow of your breath rising and falling*:

- Ever so slowly and gently, bring the delicious morsel to your lips, feeling its coolness.
- Ever so slowly and gently rub it around your lips slowly and gently around your top lip and slowly and gently around your bottom lip.
- Note any sensation – don't name it, just experience it.
- Ever so slowly lick your lips and notice the taste of the delightful and desirable flavours, its texture and aroma.
- Then gently and slowly suck the delicious juicy or creamy morsel between your soft lips and onto your tongue.
- Savour a small taste when you slowly and consciously bite gently through the juicy, juicy fruit or creamy, creamy chocolate feeling the juices and creaminess exploding in your mouth.
- Ever so slowly and ever so consciously, swallow it bit by bit.

- As you slowly savour and swallow the delicious flavours – imagine the colour of pure gold going down and down with your *Dancing Vulva Fairy* feelings – ever so slowly and gently to your stomach, then ever so slowly and gently to your vulva.
- Imagine the delicious treat on the lips of your labia majora.
- Imagine your vulva is sucking in this juicy fruit or creamy chocolate as you breathe in.
- As you breathe in, gently squeeze your thighs – now notice the delightful feeling of the juicy, juicy fruit or creamy, creamy morsel exploding within.
- Feel the delight of your *Dancing Vulva Fairy* feelings and sensations.
- Gently squeeze your pelvic floor muscles or squeeze your inner thighs together.
- Now it is time for you to breathe in the pure gold sprinkled with your *Dancing Vulva Fairy* thoughts and feelings through your vulva, then your vagina, your pelvis, your stomach and your chest – all the way up to your throat.
- Ever so slowly and gently breathe out the pure gold down to your vulva again.
- Squeeze your genital area again and imagine you are gently sucking the juicy and creamy morsel between your labia majora, your labia minora, your vagina – imagine the warmth of the pure gold and the *Dancing Vulva Fairy* thoughts and feelings moving ever so slowly up again through your pelvis, your stomach, your chest and to your throat again.
- Now, continue to focus on circulating the pure gold and the *Dancing Vulva Fairy's* tantalising energy within your body for five more times or longer if you so choose.
- Say softly to yourself: *I am comfortable, I am confident, I am in control.*
- In your own time, turn your attention to the sounds and experiences of the room and open your eyes.

You can practice this on your own while you engage in self-love through masturbation. This practice will help you to get in touch with your inner most needs and forming a deeper connection with yourself. By developing your self-awareness, it can naturally translate across when you engage in sexual activity with your partner. Something as simple as gazing into your partner's eyes is one way to begin your journey into mindful sex.

Visit *The Happy Vulva* website where you can download recordings of these exercises for your own personal use.

It's Hug Time!

Reducing Genital Image Anxiety & Rebuilding Intimacy Through Hugging

This exercise is to reintroduce hugging into your life and your partner's life. If you aren't hugging, you are both missing out on connecting. This exercise was adapted from Dr David Schnarch (1997) *Passionate Marriage: Keeping Love & Intimacy Alive in Committed Relationships*. Hugging is used to bridge emotional distance to emotional closeness and it starts *outside* the bedroom. It is designed for you to practice intimacy outside a sexual situation with your partner.

Have you noticed when your partner is wanting a hug that immediately your *Nasty Vulva Pixie* thought says:

> *Oh no! That just means he wants sex!*

Here you may avoid any physical contact with your partner. Alternatively, you may decide to have a hug and your inner *Nasty Vulva Pixie* says:

> *Oh no! This is going to turn sexual!*

Here you may end up having a stiff and awkward tree trunk hug, or you might have a quickie hug where you briefly embrace before abruptly pulling away and disengaging from your partner.

Many of us remember those long hugs and passionate kisses we used to have when we first met our partner. The intense heady feeling of having been bitten by the love bug is called *limerence*. Limerence was first coined by psychologist Dorothy Tennov in her 1979 book *Love and Limerence: The Experience of Being in Love*. Limerence is a when you have an intense sexual craving for someone. It is a feeling of euphoria. Limerence is also known as the honeymoon period of a new relationship. Limerent couples can't keep their hands off one another, they can't stop thinking about one another and their sex drive goes into overdrive. As those heady days of limerence fade, they are often replaced by the callings of domestic life and are replaced with children, careers and mortgages. Limerence was the time at the start of your love affair where Mother Nature played the bonding game. Limerence is not the barometer of what is in store in an ongoing committed relationship, as desire waxes and wanes throughout the lifespan of a couple.

Many of us find that we no longer make time for hugs in our relationship. We hug the kids, the cat or dog or our friends and relatives – but our partners are lucky if they get so much as a quick peck and a squeeze. This avoidance is not all about living a time-poor lifestyle. For many women they do not want to hug because they are worried that it might lead to sex!

Women tell me that they think that their partner only wants sex when they hug. Well, I can't argue with that – most men I have seen in my private practice nod and say 'yes', they are hoping that the hug will lead to sex. It is part of their sexual script. They expect that a hug with their sexual partner is a sure thing that will hopefully lead to sex. The hug has come to represent a part in your negative sexual script that is based on fear that it will lead to sex.

Many women notice that after practicing *It's Hug Time* they find it easier to self soothe. That they are able to tame that *Nasty Vulva Pixie*. They can enjoy the comfort of a hug with their partner without distraction. Many women say after practicing the exercise that they are more willing to engage in sexual activity with their partner.

Setting the Scene For It's Hug Time

Before you start the exercise, it is important to chat with your partner about the purpose of *It's Hug Time* as to what is going to occur and why. Explain that you will be initiating this exercise when you say *'it's hug time'* or *'let's do the hug'*. Explain to your partner that when you say *'it's hug time'* that it means an invitation to hug without the expectation that this exercise will lead to sex. It is recommended that you practice initiating the hug exercise several times a week. Practice will deepen your ability to self-soothe, while appreciating being in your partner's embrace.

To begin the hug exercise, all you and your partner have to do is to both stand on your own two feet and hug in the way you normally would. Next, let yourselves both melt into the hug and gently breathe in and out. It is important to get physically comfortable. You may need to shift around and adjust your position while maintaining physical contact with your partner as you do so.

While you are doing the exercise, make sure to notice any resistance you feel – but do not give into it and pull away. All you have to do is to continue to breathe and let your body relax, letting the resistance go away. *It's Hug Time* is not the time to be worried or wonder about what your partner is thinking or feeling or if they are having a good time or not – this is all *Nasty Vulva Pixie* talk.

If your mind wanders to such things you can return to *It's Hug Time* by using your sensory awareness of sight, sound, smell, taste and touch to centre yourself. Centering yourself involves self-soothing, turning inward and accessing your emotional tools. We engage in sensory awareness to regain a feeling of being balanced and comfortable in your body. Or if your mind wanders and your old way of thinking from the *Nasty Vulva Pixie* appears and says:

There is no time for a hug!

You can change your automatic negative thought to your new way of thinking:

There is always time for a hug!

Remember, if you persist you can move past that urge to unmerge. With practice you may even be able to relax into the physical contact and experience a feeling of comfort and closeness. If your mind wanders again, just access the skills you have leant about mindfulness, affirmations, mantras, counterstatements, distraction and visualisation.

It is important to go past that point where you want to pull away from the hug. If you notice that your partner is getting aroused by feeling the firmness of their erect penis – just notice this. For some women this is when they will pull away from the embrace. Just because he has an erection does not mean that you or he must do anything about it. It is a normal physiological reaction. Besides, it is easier to tell when your male partner is aroused, but not so obvious to notice when women are aroused. If you do pull completely away from the hug at this stage, please note what your *Nasty Vulva Pixie* is saying. If you have the urge to pull away, you can re-merge. Notice that slight discomfort and as you re-merge knowing that you can refocus again on the hug. Just notice what your *Nasty Vulva Pixie* is saying. It is important not to judge the *Nasty Vulva Pixie* thought. All you have to do is become focused on the pleasurable sights, sounds, smells, tastes, and touch that are happening through the hug again.

While you are hugging and feeling relaxed again, notice if you are experiencing any arousal sensations in your genitals, such as tingling, wetness or throbbing. Compared with men, it is harder to notice if you are aroused. Use this exercise to focus on how your body is reacting to melting into the hug. Notice if you feel turned on. It does not matter if you don't notice these feelings and sensations immediately, as it might take practice.

Here are some mantras you can employ to help drown out the *Nasty Vulva Pixie* and to bring on your *Dancing Vulva Fairy*:

- *I love a long and lingering hug.*
- *I feel safe and secure.*
- *I am connecting with myself.*
- *I am connecting with my partner.*
- *I feel loved.*
- *I feel quiet and calm.*
- *I feel connected.*
- *I am enjoying being held.*
- *I am enjoying holding my partner.*
- *Delicious, loving, giving, pleasurable, relaxing, connecting, trusting.*
- *I am feeling the electricity.*
- *I am feeling sexual vibes.*
- *My partner loves and cares for me and it is lovely to be in their arms, feeling the pressure of the hug, noticing their breath on my neck, noticing the texture of their skin or clothes.*

- *Warm, peaceful, deep, meaningful, love, tuning-in, turning-on, peace, listening to the quiet.*

You might notice your body tenses up, signalling that you want to disengage. Know that with practice it gets easier to stay in the hug. If you can, try not to abruptly pull away from the hug. You can gently say to your partner to remind them:

This is hug time.

I am enjoying just being held.

Hugs release the *cuddle chemical* called oxytocin and promote bonding and trust. Oxytocin is the love hormone that also reduces anxiety. The *It's Hug Time* exercise will assist you and your partner to melting and molding into one another, to sink gently into the experience. *Hugging* is having an emotional contact. *Not hugging* stops you from feeling connected. The added benefit of this exercise is that with practice your will learn how to have a deeper and more relaxed emotional hug. This is very different from the quickie hugs or tree trunk hugs which are stiff, awkward and create distance.

Our relationships are played out in our hugs. This exercise is about moving your experience from one of distance, to one of closeness through hugging. Moving to a more relaxing connection through the hug exercise increases the potential of you moving towards a hot and erotic connection. The good news is that all this can be achieved with your clothes on.

It's Hug Time is about learning how to hold onto and focus on yourself using your senses, breath and mindfulness to quieten yourself down. Holding onto yourself while you hold on to your partner will bring connection.

How long should the hug be? You should hold a hug until you are relaxed and then hold the hug some more. I recommend that you try for at least one minute (the longer the better) and if you can, try and hug several times a day. Some women and their partner find this exercise very moving. *It's Hug Time* is a taster of what you have been missing during sexual intimacy. *It's Hug Time* can enhance your sexual confidence and increase your sexual self-esteem. Once you have learned to make a deeper contact through your hugs you can extend this connection to sexual activity. The power of the hug can promote relaxation and calmness which can blossom into more active foreplay or outercourse.

Don't be surprised if sex takes off!

It is natural for lots of feelings to arise through this exercise – talk about the experience with your partner. You can write your feelings down about the experience, noting any barriers. If you had any *Nasty Vulva Pixies* or other automatic negative thoughts or worries. I recommend you take your concerns your next counselling and therapy session for further exploration and insights.

> *The more often you do it and the longer you do it the deeper it gets.*
>
> **– David Schnarch**

AFTERWORD

Dear *Vulva Image Warrior*

Thank you for taking the time to read *The Happy Vulva* and for embarking on this journey into and around your most private parts where you learnt many wondrous things about yourself and your body. I hope you found the experience informative and enjoyable. Please come again!

Along the way, you also learnt about the many ways that genital image anxieties exist. You delved into the cosmetic surgery industry learning about the potential risks involved in undergoing the different types of female genital cosmetic surgery. You were guided about how to raise concerns with health professionals should the need arise to discuss any genital image or sexual concerns. Finally, you explored new techniques and strategies to help you become more confident about your body and genital image in the bedroom. Your health literacy about genital image diversity and women's sexuality have increased by reading this book.

I recommend that you revisit those parts you found most helpful as well as practicing the exercises. Please share your newfound or renewed *V-Knowledge* to guide other women who may need support in this area.

Thank you again for reading *The Happy Vulva*. It has been my ambition to help increase women's genital image confidence through raising genital image diversity awareness. Please visit *The Happy Vulva* website for more information about this important area of women's sexual health where my mission will continue. I also invite you to subscribe to the *Vulva Image Warrior Movement* to receive the *V-Newsletter*.

I look forward to meeting you one day and learning about your *V-Adventures*.

– Dr Fran
Author, The Happy Vulva

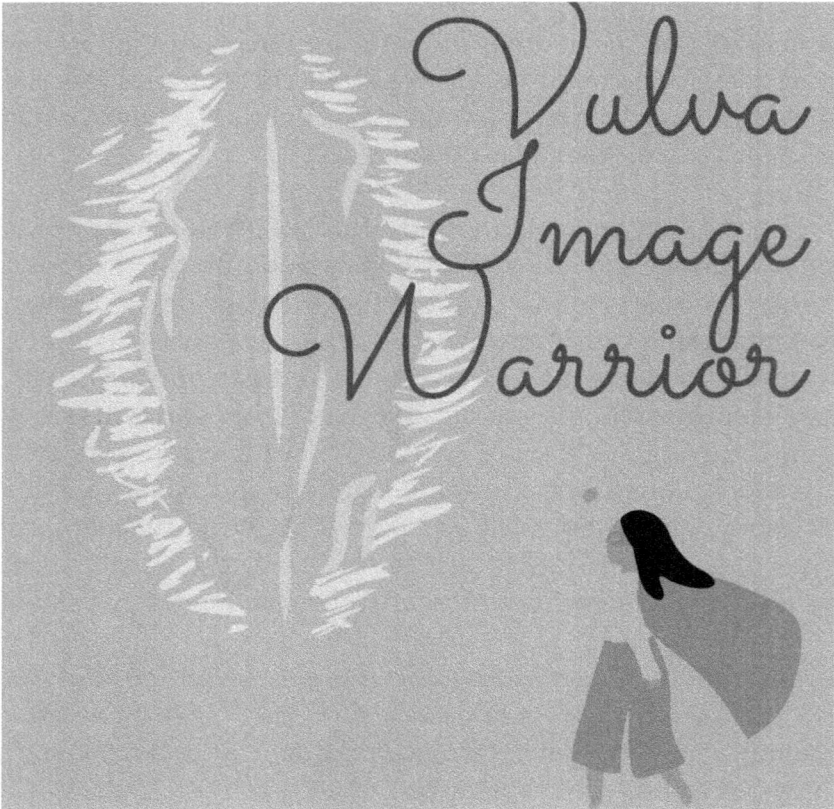

Acknowledgements

I would like to express my gratitude to the many extraordinary women who have contributed to this book. Thank you for sharing your most private thoughts and feelings about your genital image.

I am ever so grateful for the immense help and input of several wonderful and clever individuals. I would like to thank my friends and colleagues, Jane Whitmore and Brett McCann, who helped with constructive feedback and other advice. Special mention to Charmaine Morse, for reading early drafts and providing editorial help and keen insights. I am indebted to Dr Lindy McDougall for her support and taking the time to talk with me and speculate about female genital cosmetic surgery.

A huge shout-out to Kylie and Darryll Jones for the brainstorming conversations we had around the dinner table between the many Melbourne COVID-19 lockdowns. I am so appreciative for your encouragement and enthusiasm in development of the *Dancing Vulva Fairy* and *Nasty Vulva Pixie* concepts.

Thanks to everyone at *Ultimate World Publishing* who helped me so much including, Vivienne Mason and Julie Fisher. A special shout-out and thanks to Isabelle Russell for her editing prowess. Special thanks to Natasa and Stuart Denham, the ever-patient publishing manager dynamic duo. Thank you all for helping me turn my idea into a book.

To all those who have been a part of my getting there, starting with my faithful toy poodle companions, Cisco and Pancho. To Meg and Steve Kroger, Lucinda and Mark Rodrigue, Helen Nicholls-Stary and Carolina Vigars – thank you all for your gorgeous support and enthusiasm during *The Happy* Vulva process.

Finally, I would like to thank the splendid Cooper Jones. Thank you for bringing the book to life with your wondrous designs and illustrations. May your special talent prevail.

References, Resources & Other Awesome Stuff For Vulva Image Warriors

Please scan this QR code to access the links and books mentioned in *The Happy Vulva* plus:

- See the full list of resources used in the writing of *The Happy Vulva*.

- Have access to other awesome vulval resources including free audio recordings of the mindfulness exercises.

- Subscribe to the *Vulva Image Warrior Tribe* to receive the *V-Newsletter*.

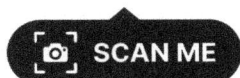

SCAN ME

About The Author

In *The Happy* Vulva, Dr Frances D'Arcy-Tehan draws upon her professional experiences with the many women she has helped during a twenty-five-year career as a counselling psychologist and sexual therapist in Australia.

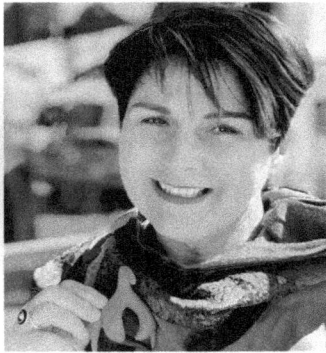

the happy vulva

_____

_____

_____

_____

_____

_____

_____

_____

_____

_____

_____

_____

_____

_____

www.ingramcontent.com/pod-product-compliance
Lightning Source LLC
Chambersburg PA
CBHW032054020426
42335CB00011B/340